INTERVENTIONAL CARDIOLOGY CLINICS

www.interventional.theclinics.com

Editor-in-Chief

MATTHEW J. PRICE

Imaging in Intervention

July 2018 • Volume 7 • Number 3

Editors

MATTHEW J. PRICE

JORGE A. GONZALEZ

ELSEVIER

1600 John F. Kennedy Boulevard • Suite 1800 • Philadelphia, Pennsylvania, 19103-2899

http://www.theclinics.com

INTERVENTIONAL CARDIOLOGY CLINICS Volume 7, Number 3
July 2018 ISSN 2211-7458, ISBN-13: 978-0-323-61297-5

Editor: Lauren Boyle
Developmental Editor: Donald Mumford

Interventional Cardiology Clinics (ISSN 2211-7458) is published quarterly by Elsevier Inc., 360 Park Avenue South, New York, NY 10010-1710. Months of issue are January, April, July, and October. Subscription prices are USD 195 per year for US individuals, USD 449 for US institutions, USD 100 per year for US students, USD 195 per year for Canadian individuals, USD 536 for Canadian institutions, USD 150 per year for Canadian students, USD 295 per year for international individuals, USD 536 for international institutions, and USD 150 per year for international students. To receive student/resident rate, orders must be accompanied by name of affiliated institution, date of term, and the *signature* of program/residency coordinator on institution letterhead. Orders will be billed at individual rate until proof of status is received. Foreign air speed delivery is included in all *Clinics* subscription prices. All prices are subject to change without notice. **POSTMASTER:** Send address changes to *Interventional Cardiology Clinics*, Elsevier Health Sciences Division, Subscription Customer Service, 3251 Riverport Lane, Maryland Heights, MO 63043. **Customer Service: Telephone: 1-800-654-2452** (U.S. and Canada); **1-314-447-8871** (outside U.S. and Canada). **Fax: 1-314-447-8029. E-mail: journalscustomerservice-usa@elsevier.com (for print support); journalsonlinesupport-usa@elsevier.com (for online support).**

Reprints. For copies of 100 or more of articles in this publication, please contact the Commercial Reprints Department, Elsevier Inc., 360 Park Avenue South, New York, NY 10010-1710. Tel.: 212-633-3874; Fax: 212-633-3820; E-mail: reprints@elsevier.com.

CONTRIBUTORS

EDITOR-IN-CHIEF

MATTHEW J. PRICE, MD
Director, Cardiac Catheterization Laboratory, Division of Cardiovascular Diseases, Scripps Clinic, Assistant Professor, Scripps Translational Science Institute, La Jolla, California, USA

EDITORS

MATTHEW J. PRICE, MD
Director, Cardiac Catheterization Laboratory, Division of Cardiovascular Diseases, Scripps Clinic, Assistant Professor, Scripps Translational Science Institute, La Jolla, California, USA

JORGE A. GONZALEZ, MD, FACC, FSCMR
Director, Advanced Cardiovascular Imaging (CT-MRI), Co-Director, Hypertrophic Cardiomyopathy Clinic, Director, Aorta Imaging Clinic, Divisions of Cardiovascular Diseases and Radiology, Scripps Clinic, La Jolla, California, USA

AUTHORS

ZIAD A. ALI, MD, DPhil
Center for Interventional Vascular Therapy, Division of Cardiology, NewYork-Presbyterian Hospital, Columbia University Irving Medical Center, Clinical Trials Center, Cardiovascular Research Foundation, New York, New York, USA; Department of Cardiology, St. Francis Hospital, Roslyn, New York, USA

MOHAMAD ALKHOULI, MD, FACC
Division of Cardiovascular Disease, Director, Structural Heart Interventions, West Virginia University School of Medicine, West Virginia University, Morgantown, West Virginia, USA

TIFFANY CHEN, MD
Advanced Cardiovascular Imaging Fellow, Department of Medicine, Cardiovascular Division, University of Pennsylvania, Philadelphia, Pennsylvania, USA

JACOB P. DAL-BIANCO, MD, FACC, FASE
Instructor in Medicine, Harvard Medical School, Heart Valve Program, Corrigan Minehan Heart Center, Massachusetts General Hospital, Boston, Massachusetts, USA

AKRAM Y. ELGENDY, MD
Cardiology Fellow, Division of Cardiovascular Medicine, Department of Medicine, University of Florida, Gainesville, Florida, USA

ISLAM Y. ELGENDY, MD, FACP, FESC
Cardiology Fellow, Division of Cardiovascular Medicine, Department of Medicine, University of Florida, Gainesville, Florida, USA

MARVIN H. ENG, MD
Structural Heart Disease Fellowship Director, Director of Research, Division of Cardiology, Center for Structural Heart Disease, Henry Ford, Detroit, Michigan, USA

VICTOR A. FERRARI, MD
Professor, Departments of Medicine and Radiology, Cardiovascular Division, University of Pennsylvania, Philadelphia, Pennsylvania, USA

T. RAYMOND FOLEY, MD
Division of Interventional Cardiology, Scripps Clinic, La Jolla, California, USA

KEYVAN KARIMI GALOUGAHI, MD, PhD
Center for Interventional Vascular Therapy, Division of Cardiology, NewYork-Presbyterian Hospital, Columbia University Irving Medical Center, New York, New York, USA

NEIL GHEEWALA, MD
Division of Cardiology, Department of
Medicine, Center for Structural Heart Disease,
Henry Ford Hospital, Detroit, Michigan, USA

MATTHEW GOTTBRECHT, MD
Department of Medicine, University of Virginia
Health System, University of Virginia,
Charlottesville, Virginia, USA

JONATHAN M. HILL, MD
London Bridge Hospital, King's College
Hospital, London, United Kingdom

HASAN JILAIHAWI, MD
Associate Professor of Medicine and
Cardiothoracic Surgery, Heart Valve Center,
NYU Langone Health, New York, New York,
USA

CHRISTOPHER M. KRAMER, MD
Division of Cardiovascular Medicine,
Department of Radiology and Medical
Imaging, Cardiovascular Imaging Center,
University of Virginia Health System,
Charlottesville, Virginia, USA

ULF LANDMESSER, MD
Department of Cardiology, Charité –
Universitätsmedizin Berlin, Berlin, Germany

JAMES C. LEE, MD
Center for Structural Heart Disease, Henry
Ford Hospital, Detroit, Michigan, USA

DMITRY LEVIN, BS
Department of Medicine, Section of
Cardiology, UW Medical Center, Seattle,
Washington, USA

ADRIÁN I. LÖFFLER, MD
Division of Cardiovascular Medicine,
University of Virginia Health System,
Charlottesville, Virginia, USA

AKIKO MAEHARA, MD
Center for Interventional Vascular Therapy,
Division of Cardiology, NewYork-Presbyterian
Hospital, Columbia University Irving Medical
Center, Clinical Trials Center, Cardiovascular
Research Foundation, New York, New York, USA

AHMED N. MAHMOUD, MD
Cardiology Fellow, Division of Cardiovascular
Medicine, Department of Medicine, University
of Florida, Gainesville, Florida, USA

DHRUV MAHTTA, MD, MBA
Resident Physician, Department of
Medicine, University of Florida, Gainesville,
Florida, USA

ROSHIN C. MATHEW, MS, MD
Department of Medicine, University of Virginia
Health System, University of Virginia,
Charlottesville, Virginia, USA

MITSUAKI MATSUMURA, BS
Clinical Trials Center, Cardiovascular Research
Foundation, New York, New York, USA

GARY S. MINTZ, MD
Clinical Trials Center, Cardiovascular Research
Foundation, New York, New York, USA

MOHAMMAD K. MOJADIDI, MD
Cardiology Fellow, Division of Cardiovascular
Medicine, Department of Medicine, University
of Florida, Gainesville, Florida, USA

ERIC MYERS, BFA
Division of Cardiology, Department of
Medicine, Center for Structural Heart Disease,
Henry Ford Hospital, Detroit, Michigan, USA

BRIAN P. O'NEILL, MD
Medical Director of TAVR Program,
Department of Medicine, Section of
Cardiology, Temple Heart and Vascular
Institute, Philadelphia, Pennsylvania, USA

WILLIAM W. O'NEILL, MD
Director, Division of Cardiology, Department
of Medicine, Center for Structural Heart
Disease, Henry Ford Hospital, Detroit,
Michigan, USA

JONATHAN J. PASSERI, MD
Assistant Professor of Medicine, Harvard
Medical School, Medical Director, Heart Valve
Program, Director of Interventional
Echocardiography, Corrigan Minehan Heart
Center, Massachusetts General Hospital,
Boston, Massachusetts, USA

HUSSEIN M. RAHIM, MD
Center for Interventional Vascular Therapy,
Division of Cardiology, NewYork-Presbyterian
Hospital, Columbia University Irving Medical
Center, New York, New York, USA

MARIANNE ROLLET, BS, RT(R)(CT)
Division of Cardiology, Department of
Medicine, Center for Structural Heart Disease,
Henry Ford Hospital, Detroit, Michigan, USA

MICHAEL SALERNO, MD, PhD
Director of Cardiac MRI, Associate
Professor of Medicine, Radiology, and BME,
Departments of Medicine, Radiology
and Medical Imaging, and Biomedical
Engineering, Cardiovascular Imaging
Center, Cardiovascular Division, University
of Virginia Health System, University
of Virginia, Charlottesville, Virginia,
USA

RAJAN SHAH, MD
Division of Cardiology, Department of
Medicine, Center for Structural Heart Disease,
Henry Ford Hospital, Detroit, Michigan,
USA

EVAN SHLOFMITZ, DO
Center for Interventional Vascular Therapy,
Division of Cardiology, NewYork-Presbyterian
Hospital, Columbia University Irving
Medical Center, Clinical Trials Center,
Cardiovascular Research Foundation, New
York, New York, USA; Department of
Cardiology, St. Francis Hospital, Roslyn,
New York, USA

RICHARD A. SHLOFMITZ, MD
Department of Cardiology, St. Francis
Hospital, Roslyn, New York, USA

FRANK E. SILVESTRY, MD, FACC, FASE
Associate Professor, Department of
Medicine, Cardiovascular Division, University
of Pennsylvania, Philadelphia, Pennsylvania,
USA

CURTISS T. STINIS, MD
Division of Interventional Cardiology, Scripps
Clinic, La Jolla, California, USA

GREGG W. STONE, MD
Center for Interventional Vascular Therapy,
Division of Cardiology, NewYork-Presbyterian
Hospital, Columbia University Irving Medical
Center, Clinical Trials Center, Cardiovascular
Research Foundation, New York, New York,
USA

ROBERT J. TALLAKSEN, MD
Department of Radiology, West Virginia
University, Morgantown, West Virginia, USA

JONATHAN M. TOBIS, MD, FACC, MSCAI
Emeritus Director of Interventional Cardiology
Research, Program in Interventional
Cardiology, Division of Cardiology, University
of California, Los Angeles, Los Angeles,
California, USA

RENU VIRMANI, MD
CVPath Institute, Gaithersburg, Maryland,
USA

DEE DEE WANG, MD
Director of Structural Heart Imaging, Medical
Director of 3D Printing Henry Ford Innovations
Institute, Division of Cardiology, Department
of Medicine, Center for Structural Heart
Disease, Henry Ford Hospital, Detroit,
Michigan, USA

MO-YANG WANG, MD
Heart Valve Center, NYU Langone Medical
Center, New York, New York, USA

LANA WINKLER, MD
Department of Radiology, West Virginia
University, Morgantown, West Virginia, USA

ZHEN-GANG ZHAO, MD
Heart Valve Center, NYU Langone Medical
Center, New York, New York, USA

CONTENTS

Intravascular imaging plays a key role in optimizing outcomes for percutaneous coronary intervention (PCI). Optical coherence tomography (OCT) uses a user-friendly interface and provides high-resolution images. OCT can be used as part of daily practice in all stages of a coronary intervention: baseline lesion assessment, stent selection, and stent optimization. Incorporating a standardized, algorithmic approach when using OCT allows for precision PCI.

Computed tomography angiography (CTA) has played a significant role in the evaluation of coronary artery disease in the last decade and has demonstrated high sensitivity and negative predictive values. However, the positive predictive value as compared with invasive fractional flow reserve (FFR) is limited. CT-FFR has emerged as a disruptive noninvasive technology with higher specificity and diagnostic accuracy for the detection of hemodynamically significant coronary lesions as compared with invasive FFR than conventional coronary CTA. CT-FFR has been shown to be cost-effective as a gate-keeper to invasive coronary angiography and has the potential to limit unnecessary invasive angiography studies.

Left ventricular dysfunction remains one of the best prognostic determinants of survival in patients with coronary artery disease. Revascularization has been shown to improve survival compared with medical therapy alone. Viability testing can help direct patients who will benefit the most from revascularization. Single-photon emission computed tomography, dobutamine stress echo, cardiac MRI, and PET imaging with F18-fluorodeoxyglucose are the most common modalities for assessing myocardial viability. Viability testing can help differentiate which patients benefit most from chronic total occlusion interventions.

Prevention of thromboembolism in atrial fibrillation has been investigated in light of the high numbers of patients unable to be treated with effective anticoagulation. Therefore, endovascular mechanical occlusion of the left atrial appendage (LAA) has been developed as a substitute for thromboprophylaxis. Initial clinical trials demonstrated high rates of procedural complications. Using computed tomography (CT), one can ascertain accurate left atrial appendage dimensions, appendage morphology; predict radiograph gantry angles; and produce physical models for ex vivo device and catheter fitting. This article is an overview of the available evidence for using CT and the clinical impact of CT on endovascular LAA occlusion.

The tricuspid valve is a highly complex structure, with variability in the number of leaflets and scallops. The mechanism of regurgitation is multifactorial in etiology, a mix of functional and degenerative tricuspid regurgitation. Iatrogenic tricuspid regurgitation is becoming more common secondary to pacemaker wire impingement of leaflet function and coaptation. Echocardiographic imaging of the tricuspid valve is particularly challenging given its anatomic location and other interfering structures, including pacemaker wires. Preprocedural planning and intraprocedural guidance for transcatheter intervention relies on a comprehensive understanding of tricuspid anatomy and the use of 3-dimensional transesophageal echocardiography. The incorporation of computed tomography and cardiac magnetic resonance imaging likely will provide increasing accuracy and optimization of procedural success.

 Video content accompanies this article at http://www.interventional.theclinics.com.

Chronic mitral regurgitation (MR), whether due to valve degeneration or secondary to myocardial disease, affects an increasing proportion of the aging population. Percutaneous mitral valve interventions, including edge-to-edge repair, are emerging as feasible and effective therapy for patients with severe MR at high or prohibitive surgical risk. Imaging with echocardiography is crucial for patient selection by evaluating mitral anatomy, the mechanism of dysfunction, and MR severity. In this article, the authors review the imaging characteristics for identifying and quantifying degenerative and functional MR for transcatheter mitral valve repair.

Rheumatic mitral stenosis remains a common disease in the developing world. Percutaneous mitral balloon valvuloplasty is an important therapy for rheumatic mitral stenosis. Echocardiography plays a critical role in the diagnosis of rheumatic mitral stenosis and the assessment of suitability for and guidance of percutaneous mitral valvuloplasty.

Three-dimensional (3D) printing is a process leading to the creation of a physical 3D model used for teaching, patient education, device evaluation, and procedural planning. 3D printed models of patient-specific anatomy can be generated from 3D transesophageal, cardiac MRI, or cardiac computed tomographic datasets. This article discusses the potential advantages of 3D printing, reviews the different modalities to acquire a 3D dataset, and highlights the application of 3D printing to enhance patient screening and procedural planning in structural heart interventions.

IMAGING IN INTERVENTION

FORTHCOMING ISSUES

October 2018
Transcatheter Aortic Valve Replacement
Susheel K. Kodali, *Editor*

January 2019
Congenital Heart Disease Intervention
Daniel S. Levi, *Editor*

April 2019
Updates in Percutaneous Coronary
Intervention
Matthew J. Price, *Editor*

RECENT ISSUES

April 2018
Left Atrial Appendage Closure
Apostolos Tzikas, *Editor*

January 2018
Transcatheter Tricuspid Valve Intervention/
Interventional Therapy for Pulmonary
Embolism
Azeem Latib and Jay Giri, *Editors*

October 2017
Transcatheter Closure of Patent Foramen
Ovale
Matthew J. Price, *Editor*

ISSUE OF RELATED INTEREST

Cardiac Electrophysiology Clinics, March 2017 (Vol. 9, Issue 1)
Ventricular Tachycardia in Structural Heart Disease
Amin Al-Ahmad and Francis E. Marchlinski, *Editors*

THE CLINICS ARE NOW AVAILABLE ONLINE!

Access your subscription at:
www.theclinics.com

PREFACE

Imaging in Intervention

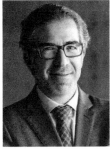 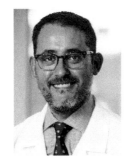

Matthew J. Price, MD   **Jorge A. Gonzalez, MD, FACC, FSCMR**
Editors

The field of cardiology has undergone increasing fragmentation in recent years. This fragmentation is manifest by the proliferation of high-level, cardiology subspecialty and subsubspecialty journals. Paradoxically, however, this hyperspecialization has led to increasing interdependence between these disciplinary silos. This interdependence is exemplified by Interventional Cardiology, in which major technological and procedural advances have bound the operator with the imager with respect to preprocedural decision making, procedural technique, and postprocedural assessment. The rapid adoption and acceptance of paradigm-shifting therapies, such as transcatheter aortic valve replacement, transcatheter mitral valve repair, and left atrial appendage closure, would not be possible without comprehensive imaging that previously would not have been considered to be part of the "wheel house" of the interventional cardiologist. This concept is not limited to the transcatheter treatment of structural heart disease: adjunctive imaging has become even more critical during percutaneous coronary intervention with the pursuit of ever-lower major adverse cardiovascular event rates and with the development of advanced techniques to treat chronic total occlusions. In the reverse direction, the development of fractional flow reserve derived from computed tomography will take concepts that are familiar to the interventionist and steer them into the realm of the noninvasive cardiologist.

This issue of *Interventional Cardiology Clinics* is dedicated to this interdisciplinary concept. Just like the theme of each article, which binds an interventional cardiology procedure with its imaging partner, this issue has been coedited by an interventional and imaging specialist. We hope that as our readers continue to subspecialize, this issue can help their path by, ironically, broadening their horizon.

Matthew J. Price, MD
Cardiac Catheterization Laboratory
Division of Cardiovascular Diseases
Scripps Clinic
9898 Genesee Avenue, AMP-200
La Jolla, CA 92037, USA

Jorge A. Gonzalez, MD, FACC, FSCMR
Advanced Cardiovascular Imaging (CT-MRI)
Hypertrophic Cardiomyopathy Clinic
Aorta Imaging Clinic
Division of Cardiovascular Diseases
Division of Radiology
Scripps Clinic
9898 Genessee Avenue
La Jolla, CA 92037, USA

E-mail addresses:
price.matthew@scrippshealth.org (M.J. Price)
gonzalez.jorge2@scrippshealth.org (J.A. Gonzalez)

Intervent Cardiol Clin 7 (2018) xi
https://doi.org/10.1016/j.iccl.2018.04.005
2211-7458/18/© 2018 Published by Elsevier Inc.

Imaging Evaluation and Interpretation for Vascular Access for Transcatheter Aortic Valve Replacement

T. Raymond Foley, MD, Curtiss T. Stinis, MD*

KEYWORDS

- Transcatheter aortic valve replacement • Vascular access • Imaging • Computed tomography
- Aortic stenosis • Sheath–to–femoral artery ratio

KEY POINTS

- Vascular access is critical to achieving successful outcomes in transcatheter aortic valve replacement (TAVR).
- Vascular complications are associated with increased mortality.
- Multidetector computed tomography (MDCT) is an important tool for assessing the aorta and peripheral vessels when planning TAVR access.
- Vessel size and calcification are risk factors for vascular complications and can be readily identified with MDCT.

INTRODUCTION

Aortic stenosis is the most common form of valvular heart disease in developed countries, affecting greater than 12% of adults over the age of 75.[1] Once symptoms develop, severe aortic stenosis is associated with greater than 50% mortality at 2 years if left untreated.[2] Over the past decade, transcatheter aortic valve replacement (TAVR) has emerged as an effective alternative to surgical intervention in patients deemed of intermediate or high surgical risk.[3–5] Additionally, TAVR has been shown to reduce hospital length of stay and cost compared with surgical aortic valve replacement.[6,7]

In many centers, TAVR is now routinely performed in a fully percutaneous fashion, obviating vascular cut-down and general anesthesia. The development of sheaths with smaller diameters has allowed for widespread adoption of this minimally invasive approach. Nonetheless, meticulous vascular access and closure remains vital to ensuring a successful procedure. Major vascular complications, which occur in a reported 11% to 16% of cases, are associated with increased hospital stay, increased cost, increased need for blood transfusions, and increased mortality.[8,9]

ACCESS SITE SELECTION

Preprocedure planning for TAVR requires a thorough vascular evaluation to determine the ideal site for vascular access. A majority of TAVR cases are currently performed in a transfemoral fashion, but inadequate vessel size and/or significant distal aortic or iliofemoral atherosclerosis may limit this approach. More than 30% of patients with critical aortic stenosis have been shown to have unfavorable iliofemoral arteries.[10] Anatomic variables that have been associated with higher rates of vascular complications include peripheral artery disease (PAD), moderate to severe iliofemoral calcification, and sheath–to–femoral artery ratio (SFAR).[8,11,12] Although not directly associated with vascular complications, severe tortuosity of the iliac vessels also should be considered when selecting an access route. Risk factors for vascular complications are listed in **Box 1**.

Division of Interventional Cardiology, Scripps Clinic, 9898 Genessee Avenue, La Jolla, CA 92037, USA
* Corresponding author.
E-mail address: stinis.curtiss@scrippshealth.org

Intervent Cardiol Clin 7 (2018) 285–291
https://doi.org/10.1016/j.iccl.2018.03.006
2211-7458/18/© 2018 Elsevier Inc. All rights reserved.

Box 1
Risk factors for vascular complications in transcatheter aortic valve replacement

Operator experience

SFAR >1.05

Moderate or severe calcification

PAD

External sheath diameter > minimal arterial diameter

Female gender

Table 1
Comparison of the clinical outcomes according to sheath–to–femoral artery ratio threshold

Variables	Sheath–to–Femoral Artery Ratio		P Value
	≥1.05 (n = 55)	<1.05 (n = 72)	
Any vascular complication	23 (41.8%)	12 (16.7%)	<.001
VARC major	17 (30.9%)	5 (6.9%)	.001
VARC minor	6 (10.9%)	7 (9.7%)	.827
Femoral artery complication	15 (27.3%)	9 (12.5%)	.035
Iliac artery complication	11 (20.0%)	2 (2.8%)	.002
In-hospital mortality	11 (20.0%)	5 (6.9%)	.033
30-d mortality	10 (18.2%)	3 (4.2%)	.016

Values are n (%). P values in bold are statistically significant.
Abbreviation: VARC, The Valve Academic Research Consortium
From Hayashida K, Lefèvre T, Chevalier B, et al. Transfemoral aortic valve implantation new criteria to predict vascular complications. JACC Cardiovasc Interv 2011;4(8):851–8; with permission.

Sheath–to–Femoral Artery Ratio

In the absence of calcified atherosclerotic disease, the common femoral artery (CFA) is able to accommodate sheaths that are slightly larger than the maximum artery diameter. In general, the femoral artery must be greater than 5.5 cm in diameter to accommodate current-generation TAVR valves.

An SFAR of greater than 1.05 has been identified as a predictor of iliofemoral vascular complications, including dissection, perforation, and rupture. Hayashida and colleagues[11] demonstrated that in 130 patients undergoing transfemoral TAVR, an SFAR greater than 1.05 was associated with a 6-fold increase in major vascular complications (30.9% vs 5.6%, P<.001), as depicted in Table 1, and significant increase in 30-day mortality (18.2% vs 2.8%, P = .004). Similarly, in a prospective registry of 137 patients undergoing transfemoral TAVR, Toggweiler and colleagues[13] demonstrated a significant increase in major and minor complications (24% vs 10%, P = .03) when external sheath diameter exceeds minimal artery diameter (Fig. 1). Furthermore, recent evidence suggests that small vessel diameters are associated with an increased risk of long-term CFA stenosis after TAVR, possibly reflecting subclinical arterial injury due to large-bore sheath insertion.[14]

It is important to distinguish between the inner diameter (ID) and outer diameter (OD) when selecting a sheath. To accurately assess SFAR, the OD should be used and consideration must be given to unexpanded and expanded OD. By convention, sheaths are standardized by their ID, and various brands of sheaths of the same ID can vary significantly with respect to their ODs. Current TAVR sheath diameters and minimal vessel requirements are listed in Table 2. The eSheath (Edwards Lifesciences LLC, Irvine, CA) has an unexpanded OD of 6.0 mm (for 20-mm, 23-mm, and 26-mm Sapien 3 valves) and 6.7 mm (for 29-mm valve); the OD increases to

7.6 mm (20-mm and 23-mm Sapien 3 valves), 8.0 mm (26-mm valve), and 8.6 mm (29-mm valve) when expanded. Similarly, the Dryseal Sheath (W. L. Gore & Associates, Flagstaff, AZ), commonly used for delivery of the Evolut R valve (Medtronic, Minneapolis, MN), has a fixed OD of 7.5 mm (for 23-mm, 26-mm, and 29-mm valves), whereas the Evolut R InLine sheath has a fixed OD of 6.0 mm (23-mm, 26-mm, and 29-mm valves) and 6.7 mm (34-mm valve). The risk of vascular injury and complications increases significantly as the sheath OD approaches vessel ID, so a proper assessment of iliofemoral access must be performed in the context of these dimensions.

Peripheral Artery Disease and Calcification

Many patients with aortic stenosis have concomitant atherosclerosis. In the PARTNER B and CoreValve ultrasound trials, 27.8% and 41.3% of patients undergoing TAVR, respectively, were found to have PAD.[4,15] Iliofemoral calcification has been shown to increase the risk of major vascular complications in transfemoral TAVR, particularly in patients with small-caliber vessels. In a prospective study of 137 patients undergoing transfemoral TAVR, Togweiller and colleagues[13] demonstrated an associated between iliofemoral calcification and vascular complications, including dissection and/or perforation of the femoral

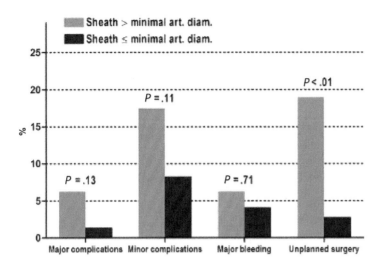

Fig. 1. Vascular complications, major bleeding, and unplanned surgery according to arterial minimal diameter and sheath external diameter as measured by iliofemoral angiography. The rate of vascular complications (major and minor combined) was higher when minimal artery diameter was smaller than the external sheath diameter (24% vs 10%, P = .03). Such patients also required more unplanned surgery. art, artery; diam, diameter; min, minimal.

artery and major bleeding. Furthermore, in a retrospective study of 19,660 patients undergoing transfemoral TAVR, the presence of PAD, regardless of degree of calcification, was associated with a significantly higher risk of vascular complications, bleeding, and death at 1 year.[12] Of particular interest for procedural planning is the presence of circumferential and/or horseshoe calcification, which limits arterial compliance and increases the risk of dissection and perforation with sheath insertion.

Vessel Tortuosity

Iliofemoral tortuosity has important implications for TAVR access. Although not clearly associated with vascular complications, severe angulation (eg, >90°) is a relative contraindication to large-bore access. Sheath advancement is challenging in the presence of significant tortuosity and may predispose to dissection, perforation, sheath kinking, and difficulty with valve delivery, even if stiff wires are used. Importantly, circumferential calcification located within tortuous segments should not be expected to straighten with stiff guide wires due to inflexibility of the vessel, and this can be an impediment to sheath and valve system delivery even if the ID of the vessel appears large enough for safe device passage.

Table 2
Sheath dimensions and minimal vessel requirements for Edwards and Medtronic valves

Edwards Sapien 3	Transcatheter Heart Valve	eSheath Outer Diameter (Unexpanded)	Maximum eSheath Outer Diameter (Expanded with Crimped Transcatheter Heart Valve)	Minimum Vessel Required (1:1.05 Sheath:Artery)
	20 mm	—	—	—
	23 mm	6 mm	7.6 mm	7.2 mm
	26 mm	6 mm	8 mm	7.6 mm
	29 mm	6.7 mm	8.6 mm	8.2 mm
Medtronic Evolut R	Transcatheter Heart Valve	Sheath Outer Diameter		Minimum Vessel Required (1:1.05 sheath:artery)
	23 mm	6 mm		5.7 mm
	26 mm	6 mm		5.7 mm
	29 mm	6 mm		5.7 mm
	31 mm	6.8 mm		6.5 mm

COMPUTED TOMOGRAPHY

MDCT has emerged as the gold standard for vascular assessment prior to TAVR. MDCT provides a comprehensive, 3-D assessment of ileofemoral and thoracic vascular anatomy, including the minimal luminal area of the femoral arteries and the presence of extreme tortuosity, calcification, aneurysmal disease, and dissections. MDCT can also identify the presence of aortic atheroma, which may pose an obstacle to valve advancement and increase the risk of cerebral or distal embolization.

Image acquisition should be performed using an MDCT scanner with a least 64 detectors. Nongated spiral acquisition can be performed to limit radiation exposure, but the prevalence of cardiac arrhythmias in the population often necessitates retrospective gating to enhance image reconstruction. A complete study should assess the entire aorta as well as iliofemoral, subclavian, and apical access routes. The latter 2 sites require ECG gating to limit motion artifact and improve temporal resolution. Importantly, imaging of the axillary and subclavian arteries should be performed with the arms positioned alongside the body to prevent pseudostenosis in the acquired images.[16]

Standard acquisitions are demonstrated in **Fig. 2**. Peripheral access is assessed using curved multiplanar reconstruction (MPR) and 3-D volume-rendered images.

At the authors' institution, the CT report includes (1) minimal internal diameter of the abdominal aorta as well as bilateral common iliac, external iliac, femoral and subclavian arteries, (2) qualitative description of vessel tortuosity, and (3) qualitative description of presence and degree of calcification and atherosclerotic plaque. It is imperative for the TAVR operators to review the MDCT images in detail themselves to gain a comprehensive understanding of the patient's vascular anatomy prior to TAVR. At the authors' institution, this is performed in a multidisciplinary setting with the input of interventional cardiologists, general cardiologists, cardiothoracic surgeons, and radiologists.

Low-Contrast Protocols

Standard MDCT for TAVR planning uses between 100 mL and 120 mL of intravenous contrast. In patients with renal impairment, low-contrast protocols can be used to successfully obtain the necessary imaging while minimizing the risk of contrast-induced nephropathy. Pulwerwitz and colleagues[17] demonstrated successful (96% diagnostic accuracy) pre-TAVR CTA imaging in 26 patients with chronic kidney disease and estimated glomerular filtration rates less than 30 mL/min using a novel very-low-contrast volume with 20 µL of iodinated contrast. Similarly, Kok and colleagues[18] have described the successful use of a 40-µL protocol in obtaining sufficient diagnostic quality images for pre-TAVR assessment.

At the authors' institution, a standard pre-TAVR CTA is performed using 100 µL of contrast. For patients with significant renal impairment (eg, glomerular filtration rate <30 mL/min), the authors use a low-contrast

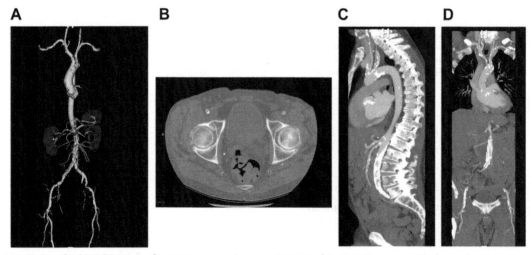

Fig. 2. Standard MDCT images for TAVR access planning. CTA (*A*) of the entire aorta and iliofemoral system demonstrates severe calcification in the distal aorta and iliacs bilaterally. The transverse plane (*B*) is most useful for assessing femoral calcification. The coronal plane (*D*) allows for an assessment of tortuosity, whereas the sagittal view (*C*) demonstrates diffuse calcification in the distal aorta.

protocol that allows for adequate imaging with less than 40 μL of contrast.

INVASIVE ANGIOGRAPHY

Conventional iliofemoral angiography can be used to assess the patency of the distal aorta, common and external iliac arteries, and the femoral arteries prior to TAVR. This method can be conveniently performed at the time of coronary angiography with a pigtail catheter, calibrated to facilitate minimal luminal diameter assessment, and minimal contrast. Despite excellent spatial resolution, angiography provides a 2-D assessment lacking orthogonal views. As a result, accurate luminal areas cannot be obtained with angiography alone. In a study of 496 patients undergoing transfemoral TAVR, contrast CT was found superior to angiography in predicting risk of vascular complications.[19]

MAGNETIC RESONANCE ANGIOGRAPHY

Magnetic resonance angiography (MRA) has been proposed as an alternative to CTA for TAVR planning in select patients. Although the use of gadolinium is contraindicated in patients with severe renal dysfunction due to the risk for nephrogenic systemic fibrosis, MRA with ferumoxytol contrast has been successfully used to obtain ilifemoral dimensions in patients with renal impairment.[20] Ruile and colleagues[21] recently described the use of noncontrast MRA in pre-TAVR vascular access planning and found that diagnostic quality was comparable to CTA.

INTRAVASCULAR ULTRASOUND

Intravascular ultrasound provides a high-resolution, 3-D assessment of vessel size as well as plaque burden and composition. This is an invasive modality that may be used to assess vessel dimensions prior to TAVR in select cases (eg, poor renal function). This technique has been described for graft planning in endovascular aortic aneurysm repair, but few data currently exist pertaining to TAVR access.[22,23]

OBTAINING FEMORAL ACCESS

Femoral access for interventions requiring large-bore sheaths should be obtained with a single, front wall puncture to minimize the risk of complications. The arteriotomy should be located in the CFA below the inguinal ligament, proximal to the bifurcation of the superficial femoral and profunda femoris arteries and superficial to the ilio-pubic eminence to provide an area for manual

compression during sheath removal and Perclose ProGlide devices (Abbott Vascular, Santa Clara, CA). In addition to anatomic landmarks, a variety of imaging modalities can be used to enhance the precision of vascular access. These include fluoroscopy, ultrasound, and angiography.

Fluoroscopy

Fluoroscopy should be used to confirm that vascular access is obtained at the level of the ilio-pubic eminence (see **Fig. 1**). A brief fluoroscopic image can be obtained with the index and second finger positioned on the femoral pulse to allow for direct visualization of the CFA in relationship to the bony structures. At the authors' institution, femoral access for TAVR is obtained using fluoroscopy and femoral angiography from a contralateral access point (see **Fig. 2**). This technique allows for direct visualization of the femoral artery and anatomic landmarks during vascular access.

Ultrasound

Ultrasound can be a useful adjunct in defining the course of the femoral artery and identifying the bifurcation of the superficial femoral and profunda femoris arteries if ambiguity remains despite a careful review of MDCT images. Ultrasound has been shown to improve CFA cannulation in patients with high bifurcations and to reduce the time and number of attempts necessary to obtain arterial access compared with fluoroscopy alone.[24] Ultrasound-guided femoral access has also been associated with a significant reduction postprocedure hematoma formation.[25]

For TAVR access, direct visualization with ultrasound may allow the operator to avoid puncturing the artery in a site of heavy calcific plaque, which may compromise percutaneous closure. Importantly, ultrasound must be used in conjunction with fluoroscopic bony landmarks to avoid a high stick (eg, above the inguinal ligament) and the associated risk of retroperitoneal hemorrhage.

ALTERNATIVE ACCESS SITES

In patients with inadequate femoral access due to calcified atherosclerotic disease, excessive tortuosity, or a high bifurcation, alternative sites for access must be considered. Alternatives to femoral access include subclavian, direct aortic, transapical, transcarotid, and transcaval. Although feasible, these approaches are associated with higher rates of complications and mortality due to the prevalence of comorbidities and less operator experience. Importantly, having access to and experience with more than 1 TAVR system (e.g., Edwards Sapien S3 and Medtronic Evolut R) allows for more options for treating patients and often obviates performing more challenging alternative access scenarios, such as transcaval, direct aortic, transapical, and transcarotid.

CLOSURE

Femoral

The most common closure technique for percutaneous transfemoral TAVR is the "pre-close" method. This technique uses sequential deployment of 2 Perclose ProGlide devices (Abbott Vascular, Santa Clara, CA) in a crosshair approach (10 o'clock and 2 o'clock positions).[26] Hemostasis is dependent on the successful delivery and positioning of monofilament polypropylene suture to the arteriotomy. Extensive anterior calcification has the potential to compromise suture delivery and is a relative contraindication to use of the "pre-close" technique. In some cases, pre-TAVR CT and US guidance may allow an operator to identify an area free of calcium and appropriate for suture-mediated hemostasis. In cases where a calcium-free zone cannot be identified, alternative access or direct femoral cut down and repair should be pursued.

SUMMARY

TAVR is a safe and effective therapy for severe aortic stenosis. Successful vascular access and closure are critical to achieving optimal outcomes and require a careful preprocedure assessment of vascular anatomy. Circumferential calcification and small-caliber vessels increase the risk of vascular complication, which are associated with increased morbidity, mortality, and cost. MDCT provides high-resolution, 3-D imaging and is considered the gold standard for access planning in TAVR. As the clinical applications of TAVR continue to expand, the imaging evaluation and interpretation of peripheral vasculature will remain an essential skill in structural intervention.

REFERENCES

1. Osnabrugge RLJ, Mylotte D, Head SJ, et al. Aortic stenosis in the elderly: disease prevalence and number of candidates for transcatheter aortic valve replacement: a meta-analysis and modeling study. J Am Coll Cardiol 2013;62(11):1002–12.
2. Freeman RV, Otto CM. Spectrum of calcific aortic valve disease: pathogenesis, disease progression, and treatment strategies. Circulation 2005;111(24):3316–26.
3. Leon MB, Smith CR, Mack MJ, et al. Transcatheter or surgical aortic-valve replacement in intermediate-risk patients. N Engl J Med 2016;374(17):1609–20.
4. Leon MB, Smith CR, Mack M, et al. Transcatheter aortic-valve implantation for aortic stenosis in patients who cannot undergo surgery. N Engl J Med 2010;363(17):1597–607.
5. Reardon MJ, Van Mieghem NM, Popma JJ, et al. Surgical or transcatheter aortic-valve replacement in intermediate-risk patients. N Engl J Med 2017;376(14):1321–31.
6. Cohen DJ. Cost-effectiveness of trancatheter vs. surgical aortic valve replacement in intermediate risk patients: results from the PARTNER 2A and Sapien 3 intermediate risk trials. Presented at: TCT 2017. Denver, CO, October 31, 2017.
7. Burrage M, Moore P, Cole C, et al. Transcatheter aortic valve replacement is associated with comparable clinical outcomes to open aortic valve surgery but with a reduced length of in-patient hospital stay: a systematic review and meta-analysis of randomised trials. Heart Lung Circ 2017;26(3):285–95.
8. Sardar MR, Goldsweig AM, Abbott JD, et al. Vascular complications associated with transcatheter aortic valve replacement. Vasc Med 2017;22(3):234–44.
9. Généreux P, Webb JG, Svensson LG, et al. Vascular complications after transcatheter aortic valve replacement: insights from the PARTNER (Placement of AoRTic TraNscathetER Valve) trial. J Am Coll Cardiol 2012;60(12):1043–52.
10. Kurra V, Schoenhagen P, Roselli EE, et al. Prevalence of significant peripheral artery disease in patients evaluated for percutaneous aortic valve insertion: preprocedural assessment with multidetector computed tomography. J Thorac Cardiovasc Surg 2009;137(5):1258–64.
11. Hayashida K, Lefèvre T, Chevalier B, et al. Transfemoral aortic valve implantation new criteria to predict vascular complications. JACC Cardiovasc Interv 2011;4(8):851–8.
12. Fanaroff AC, Manandhar P, Holmes DR, et al. Peripheral artery disease and transcatheter aortic valve replacement outcomes: a report from the society of thoracic surgeons/American college of cardiology transcatheter therapy registry. Circ Cardiovasc Interv 2017;10(10). https://doi.org/10.1161/CIRCINTERVENTIONS.117.005456.
13. Toggweiler S, Gurvitch R, Leipsic J, et al. Percutaneous aortic valve replacement: vascular outcomes with a fully percutaneous procedure. J Am Coll Cardiol 2012;59(2):113–8.
14. Shoeib O, Burzotta F, Aurigemma C, et al. Percutaneous transcatheter aortic valve replacement

induces femoral artery shrinkage: angiographic evidence and predictors for a new side effect. Catheter Cardiovasc Interv 2017. https://doi.org/10.1002/ccd.27248.

15. Adams DH, Popma JJ, Reardon MJ, et al. Transcatheter aortic-valve replacement with a self-expanding prosthesis. N Engl J Med 2014; 370(19):1790–8.

16. Litmanovich DE, Ghersin E, Burke DA, et al. Imaging in Transcatheter Aortic Valve Replacement (TAVR): role of the radiologist. Insights Imaging 2014;5(1):123–45.

17. Pulerwitz TC, Khalique OK, Nazif TN, et al. Very low intravenous contrast volume protocol for computed tomography angiography providing comprehensive cardiac and vascular assessment prior to transcatheter aortic valve replacement in patients with chronic kidney disease. J Cardiovasc Comput Tomogr 2016;10(4):316–21.

18. Kok M, Turek J, Mihl C, et al. Low contrast media volume in pre-TAVI CT examinations. Eur Radiol 2016;26(8):2426–35.

19. Okuyama K, Jilaihawi H, Kashif M, et al. Transfemoral access assessment for transcatheter aortic valve replacement: evidence-based application of computed tomography over invasive angiography. Circ Cardiovasc Imaging 2015;8(1). https://doi.org/10.1161/CIRCIMAGING.114.001995.

20. Kallianos K, Henry TS, Yeghiazarians Y, et al. Ferumoxytol MRA for transcatheter aortic valve replacement planning with renal insufficiency. Int J Cardiol 2017;231:255–7.

21. Ruile P, Blanke P, Krauss T, et al. Pre-procedural assessment of aortic annulus dimensions for transcatheter aortic valve replacement: comparison of a non-contrast 3D MRA protocol with contrast-enhanced cardiac dual-source CT angiography. Eur Heart J Cardiovasc Imaging 2016;17(4):458–66.

22. White RA, Donayre C, Kopchok G, et al. Intravascular ultrasound: the ultimate tool for abdominal aortic aneurysm assessment and endovascular graft delivery. J Endovasc Surg 1997;4(1):45–55.

23. Slovut DP, Ofstein LC, Bacharach JM. Endoluminal AAA repair using intravascular ultrasound for graft planning and deployment: a 2-year community-based experience. J Endovasc Ther 2003;10(3):463–75.

24. Seto AH, Abu-Fadel MS, Sparling JM, et al. Real-time ultrasound guidance facilitates femoral arterial access and reduces vascular complications: FAUST (Femoral Arterial Access With Ultrasound Trial). JACC Cardiovasc Interv 2010; 3(7):751–8.

25. Kalish J, Eslami M, Gillespie D, et al. Routine use of ultrasound guidance in femoral arterial access for peripheral vascular intervention decreases groin hematoma rates. J Vasc Surg 2015;61(5):1231–8.

26. Barbash IM, Barbanti M, Webb J, et al. Comparison of vascular closure devices for access site closure after transfemoral aortic valve implantation. Eur Heart J 2015;36(47):3370–9.

Imaging Evaluation for the Detection of Leaflet Thrombosis After Transcatheter Aortic Valve Replacement

Zhen-Gang Zhao, MD, Mo-Yang Wang, MD,
Hasan Jilaihawi, MD*

KEYWORDS

- Transcatheter aortic valve replacement • Leaflet thrombosis • Hypoattenuated leaflet thickening
- Reduced leaflet motion • Hypoattenuation affecting motion

KEY POINTS

- On contrast computed tomography (CT) views, hypoattenuated leaflet thickening (HALT) may be visible as wedge-shaped or semilunar opacities in both systole and diastole.
- The presence of HALT prompts the need for an assessment of reduced leaflet motion (RELM) using 4-D VR CT. The view with maximal leaflet opening is identified to assess RELM severity, expressed as the percentage of actual to expected opening and graded as mild (<50%), moderate (50% to 69%), severe (70% to 99%), and immobile.
- HALT with significant RELM (>50%), specifically described as hypoattenuation affecting motion, formed the bases of the definition for subclinical leaflet thrombosis.
- If CT evaluation is not feasible, transesophageal echocardiography may serve as an alternative imaging modality for the detection of leaflet thrombosis, given the excellent concordance between the 2 modalities.

INTRODUCTION

With the expansion of transcatheter aortic valve replacement (TAVR) into younger and lower-risk patient populations, valve durability has become a more relevant issue that draws increasing attention. Leaflet thrombosis has thus been an increased focus of attention and presents as a spectrum (Fig. 1); it may be (1) clinical (when the patient presents post-TAVR with embolic symptoms or dyspnea/chest pain, commonly but not always with elevated gradients); (2) subclinical with hemodynamic sequelae (elevated gradients on routine echocardiography without symptoms); or (3) entirely subclinical (no symptoms or hemodynamic or embolic sequelae). Although the first 2 categories are rare and the hemodynamic performance of TAVR bioprostheses have been noted to be superior to surgical bioprostheses at follow-up to 5 years and beyond,[1] recent studies based on 3-D or 4-D volume-rendered (VR) computed tomography (CT) have reported a higher prevalence of subclinical (generally without hemodynamic sequelae) hypoattenuated leaflet thickening (HALT) with or without reduced leaflet motion (RELM) of TAVR than surgical bioprostheses.[2–8] This common imaging finding has raised concerns over TAVR valve durability and

Conflicts of Interest: Dr H. Jilaihawi is a consultant for Edwards Lifesciences and Venus Medtech. The other authors have no relationships relevant to the contents of this article to disclose.
Heart Valve Center, New York University Langone Health, 530 1st Avenue, Suite 9V, New York, NY 10016, USA
* Corresponding author. Heart Valve Center, New York University Langone Health, 530 1st Avenue, Suite 9V, New York, NY 10016.
E-mail address: hasanjilaihawi@gmail.com

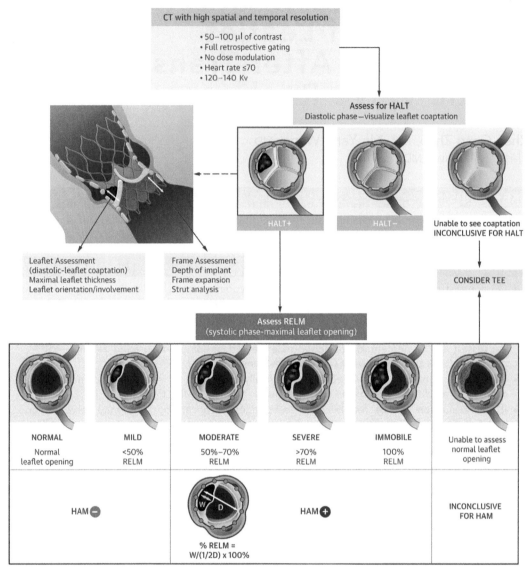

Fig. 1. CT evaluation of leaflet thrombosis. (*Top*) HALT is assessed in a diastolic phase with visualization of leaflet coaptation required for a conclusive scan. There is an additional assessment of the valve leaflets in the presence of HALT in the diastolic phase. In the presence of HALT, RELM is quantified in a systolic phase with a VR en face projection (*bottom*) at maximal leaflet opening (see **Fig. 2**). Moderate, severe, or leaflet immobility on RELM analysis in the presence of HALT is described as HAM. With inconclusive HALT (or HAM), TEE may be considered. (*From* Jilaihawi H, Asch FM, Manasse E, et al. Systematic CT methodology for the evaluation of subclinical leaflet thrombosis. JACC Cardiovasc Imaging 2017;10(4):463; with permission.)

debates on optimal postprocedural antiplatelet/anticoagulation regime.[9]

Up to now, the long-term hemodynamic consequences and clinical impact of subclinical leaflet thrombosis have remained unclear. This article describes a systematic CT imaging methodology used for the evaluation of leaflet thrombosis after TAVR,[10] which may help gather standardized and valuable information for a better understanding of the phenomenon.

OPTIMAL TIMING FOR THE DETECTION OF SUBCLINICAL LEAFLET THROMBOSIS

The optimal timing of CT scan for the detection of subclinical leaflet thrombosis remains unknown, in view of the current knowledge that the period during which the phenomenon may start to develop is not restricted to a brief window after the procedure but may develop over a prolonged period. In the Subclinical Aortic Valve Bioprosthesis Thrombosis Assessed with 4D Computed Tomography (SAVORY) registry, the interval between TAVR or surgical aortic valve replacement (SAVR) and the development of HALT was highly variable.[8] In this study, CT scans obtained at different time points within the first year after TAVR or SAVR detected HALT and hypoattenuation affecting motion (HAM) in approximately 40% and 20% of the patients, respectively.[8] The earliest scan showing HALT was performed 21 days after TAVR, indicating that HALT could develop very early after the procedure.[8] Similarly, another study observed HALT in 10% of the patients on CT scans performed at a median interval of 5 days after TAVR.[3] Further investigations with larger sample sizes and prolonged follow-up are warranted so as to seek a better understanding of the natural history of HALT and RELM and help determine the best timing of a CT scan for the detection of leaflet thrombosis and follow-up.

COMPUTED TOMOGRAPHY ACQUISITION PROTOCOLS

Adequate CT imaging quality is a necessity for the visualization and precise evaluation of leaflet hypoattenuation and motion. Although there is currently no specifically recommended protocol, there are some general principles that could be followed to obtain interpretable CT images for this purpose.

- Scans must be contrast enhanced. The optimal amount of contrast medium depends on the scanner but is approximately 50 mL to 100 mL. Because renal function is usually a concern for TAVR patients, however, the volume of contrast should be adjusted according to each patient's renal function to reduce the risk of contrast-induced nephropathy. In the authors' practice, the minimal contrast volume used is 50 mL and the upper limit is set individually for each patient at twice the numerical creatinine clearance in milliliters per minute. This practice is primarily based on the experiences from acute kidney injury in percutaneous coronary intervention studies.[11,12]
- Full retrospective gating is required to enable the creation of 4-D animations for the assessment of leaflet motion throughout the cardiac cycle.
- Scan slice thickness should be submillimeter.

- A CT scanner with the highest resolution available should be used.
- Dose modulation preferably should not be used.
- Heart rate reduction with β-blockade should be considered if resting heart rate is above 70 beats/min to minimize the possibility of artifact, particularly in patients with atrial fibrillation.
- The standard scanner acquisition voltage of 120 kV is usually adequate. A higher voltage of 140 kV may bring some additional benefits, especially in situations discussed later, but may be at the cost of contrast delineation of hypoattenuation; 140 kV also increases the dose of radiation and the field of scan should thus be limited to the prosthesis alone.
  ○ A large body habitus
  ○ A denser bioprosthetic stent frame, such as the Lotus valve (Boston Scientific, Natick, Massachusetts) or an earlier-generation CoreValve (Medtronic, Minneapolis, Minnesota) or Sapien or Sapien XT (Edwards Lifesciences, Irvine, California) prosthesis
  ○ Additional intracardiac devices, such as pacemaker leads
  ○ Coexisting mechanical or bioprosthetic valves (including TAVR valve-in-valve)

COMPUTED TOMOGRAPHY TECHNICAL QUALITY

Technical quality is the basis of standardized assessment and reporting of subclinical leaflet thrombosis. A quality score has been developed for this purpose and described previously.[10] The quality scoring system takes into consideration the varying stent frame density of different bioprostheses that could generate varying degrees of artifact. As discussed previously, the Lotus valve, Sapien/Sapien XT valve, and earlier-generation CoreValve are the densest and may generate the most artifacts. In contrast, a valve, such as the Portico valve (St. Jude Medical, Minneapolis, MN), has thin struts and as a result much less artifact on CT images. Similarly, most surgical bioprostheses have little metal material in their frames and produce little artifact. These are observations based primarily on the observation over several studies, including Portico trial, Assessment of TRanscathetEr and Surgical Aortic BiOprosthetic Valve Thrombosis and Its TrEatment With Anticoagulation (RESOLVE), and SAVORY registries and remain to be confirmed in future systematic comparative studies.

To definitively exclude subclinical leaflet thrombosis, the scan quality should allow clear visualization of central leaflet coaptation coupled with the absence of hypoattenuation associated with leaflets. This could be assessed in a cross-sectional 2-D multiplanar reconstruction (MPR)/axial view. If hypoattenuated material is observed on a 2-D view, additional evaluation of leaflet motion with the use of 4-D CT should be performed to quantify the severity. According the quality scoring system, the minimal quality requirement of a CT scan used for quantifying the severity of RELM should be at least "good." A scan with borderline quality can at most determine the presence or absence of leaflet-associated hypoattenuation.

In reporting a subclinical leaflet thrombosis, the conclusion that could be made may fall into one of the following categories:

- HALT is absent and HAM-negative per definition, thereby there is no need for RELM assessment (scan quality borderline to excellent).
- HALT is present, thus prompting the need for further assessment of RELM (scan with good to excellent quality is required to determine the severity of RELM).
- HALT is indeterminate (scan quality poor or very poor).

If HALT is present, severity of RELM may be graded on further evaluation as

- Significantly reduced ($\geq$50% reduction) and thus by definition HAM-positive
- Not significantly reduced (<50% reduction) and hence HAM-negative (scan quality good to excellent)
- Indeterminate (scan quality poor, very poor, or borderline)

Although this framework is empirical, it offers a clear definition for reporting that enables further study and collaboration.

If CT evaluation is not feasible owing to contraindication or limited scan quality, transesophageal echocardiography (TEE) may serve as an alternative imaging modality for the detection of leaflet thrombosis, given the excellent concordance between the 2 modalities with respect to the visualization of leaflet thickening and mobility.[2]

COMPUTED TOMOGRAPHY ANALYSIS SOFTWARE AND PROTOCOLS

All commercially available workstations could be used for the assessment of HALT in a diastolic-phase 2-D MPR view. For the evaluation of leaflet motion and grading of RELM based on the systematic methodology introduced in this article, however, the software used should be capable of reconstructing multiphase 3-D VR images throughout the cardiac cycle to generate 4-D VR images. There are multiple imaging postprocessing software programs broadly available for generating 4-D animations, including the 3mensio Valves (Pie Medical Imaging BV, Bilthoven, The Netherlands), Vitrea software (Vital Images, Minnetonka, Minnesota), and several others.

For the detection of HALT, 2-D axial cross-sectional MPR and 3-D VR images are used to assess the valve leaflets systematically. To acquire a clear visualization of the leaflets and minimize the interference of artifacts, the window level usually needs to be adjusted individually for each patient. If HALT is noted during the evaluation of leaflet morphology, then 3-D VR images should be generated throughout the cardiac cycle to obtain an animation movie of the bioprosthetic valve (4-D VR CT). Further analysis is then focused on the detection of leaflet motion abnormality and quantification of its severity on the frame with maximal valve opening according to the aforementioned cutoffs and definitions.

Although it is challenging to get a clear visualization of leaflets with normal thickness and motion on 4-D VR CT, thickened leaflets with reduced motion are generally clearly seen in 3-D or 4-D images providing that the image quality is reasonable.

HYPOATTENUATED LEAFLET THICKENING

Normally, bioprosthetic leaflets of all types of TAVR devices are very thin and may be barely visible even on high-quality CT scans. HALT, which refers to hypoattenuation associated with bioprosthetic leaflets observed on CT images, is the hallmark of subclinical leaflet thrombosis, particularly when seen early after TAVR. On 2-D longitudinal views, abnormal leaflets appear as thick hypodense lines, which are always thickest at the periphery or base of the leaflets and tapered toward the free edges of the leaflet. On axial views, abnormal leaflets may be visible as wedge-shaped or semilunar opacities in both systolic and diastolic phases (see Fig. 1; Fig. 2). There is considerable interindividual variability with respect to the degree of involvement of the hypoattenuating lesions, with

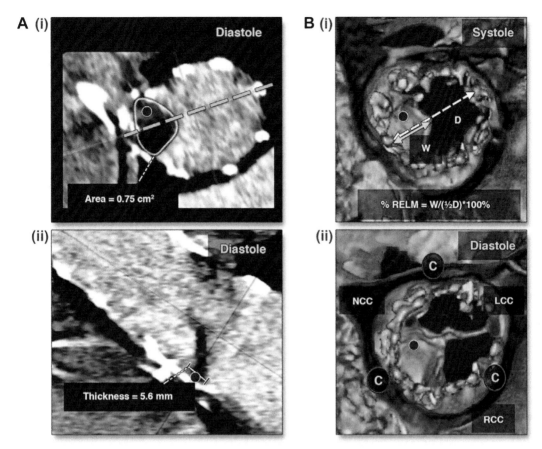

Fig. 2. Appearance and evaluation of leaflet thrombosis. Shown as characteristic wedge-shaped or semilunar opacities in the form of HALT. (*A* [*i*]) 2-D axial MPR; (*A* [*ii*]) corresponding 2-D longitudinal MPR (derived from *green dashed line* [*A* (*i*)]); (*B*) 3-D en face VR projection in both systole (maximal leaflet opening) (*B* [*i*]) and diastole (*B* [*ii*]) (clear coaptation should be seen, generally 80% used). Efforts to quantify HALT include measurement of maximal area for each leaflet affected (*A* [*i*]) and maximal thickness (*B* [*ii*]); volumetric methods also may be used. A further quantitative parameter of %RELM also may be used as [a = W/(1/2D) * 100%], where, on a 3-D en face VR projection during maximal leaflet opening, W is the base-to-tip width and D is the diameter within the stent frame (*B* [*i*]). A %RELM greater than 50% denotes HAM. The orientation of the affected bioprosthetic leaflet(s) (*B* [*ii*] *red dot*) is designated in relation to the native commissures (*C*) and sinuses. LCC, left coronary cusp; NCC, noncoronary cusp; RCC, right coronary cusp. (*From* Jilaihawi H, Asch FM, Manasse E, et al. Systematic CT methodology for the evaluation of subclinical leaflet thrombosis. JACC Cardiovasc Imaging 2017;10(4):465; with permission.)

a wide variation in leaflet thickness and reduction in motion.

TEE has been the gold standard imaging modality for the evaluation of valve leaflet structure and function. In a previous attempt to validate the use of CT imaging for the assessment of HALT and RELM through blinded analysis in 10 patients from the Portico trial, a complete correlation was noted between CT and TEE in terms of the range of lesion involvement and its morphology.[2] On TEE, abnormal bioprosthetic leaflets were shown to be covered with hyperechogenic and homogeneous mass on the aortic surface with a clearly delineated contour. This echocardiographic pattern is in complete agreement with the CT imaging findings, as described previously.

In the presence of relatively denser stent frame, such as that of the Lotus or an earlier-generation CoreValve, or Sapien or Sapien XT prosthesis, there could be considerable artifact on CT images that may obscure a clear delineation of leaflet structure, if only a single phase is acquired. In such settings, the availability of multiphase CT images with retrospective gating will enable the clarification of artifacts, which may be present only in a single phase. Moreover, only with multiphase images is it possible to assess leaflet motion throughout the cardiac cycle (see **Fig. 2**).

REDUCED LEAFLET MOTION AND HYPOATTENUATION AFFECTING MOTION

Maximal leaflet excursion can be assessed with the use of 4-D VR en face CT images of the aortic bioprosthesis. The phase with maximal leaflet excursion should be identified for further delicate measurements and quantification. The distance between the inner margin of the frame and the maximally open leaflet tip of the most affected leaflet is taken as the numerator (leaflet width [W]); the distance between the frame margin and its center, or half of the frame diameter, is taken as the denominator (1/2D). The percentage of reduction in leaflet motion (%RELM) is thereby calculated using the formula: [%RELM = W/(1/2D) * 100%] (see **Fig. 1**).

In turn, the severity of RELM could then be categorized as normal, mild (<50% reduction of leaflet motion), moderate (50% to 69% reduction), severe (70% to 99% reduction), and immobile (in at least 1 of the leaflets). It should be acknowledged, however, that the present temporal resolution of CT (at ≥70 ms for the most technically capable scanners) may diminish the accuracy of such strata.

Empirically, mild RELM (<50% reduction) was defined as nonsignificant whereas more-than-mild RELM (≥50% reduction) was considered significant (see **Figs. 1** and **2**). The presence of significant RELM was used in our practice as the standardized threshold for the discrimination between the potentially pathologic phenomenon of subclinical leaflet thrombosis and the likely physiologic thin layer of leaflet hypoattenuation, which may be associated with the adherence of fibrin. The latter could be observed on SAVR or TAVR bioprosthetic leaflets with contrast CT shortly after the procedure, particularly with very-high-quality scans.

The coexistence of the 2 phenomena, HALT and significant RELM (≥50% reduction in leaflet motion) as seen on 4-D CT, formed the bases of the definition for subclinical leaflet thrombosis used in the Portico, RESOLVE, and SAVORY studies, which has been specifically described as HAM.

LEAFLET THICKNESS AND THROMBUS BURDEN

Leaflet thickness can be measured on a 2-D diastolic-phase longitudinal MPR view showing the maximal leaflet thickness. This view could be obtained by aligning the crosshairs in a cross-sectional MPR projection and thus generating a corresponding longitudinal view cutting through the middle of the affected leaflet. Accurate positioning of the crosshair allows more reliable comparison with subsequent follow-up scans to determine the progression or regression of HALT and also enables the comparison between different studies.

Alternatively, and as a supplementary index for the quantitative assessment of thrombus burden, maximal HALT area may be defined and measured on an axial cross-sectional view, which shows the largest range of HALT involvement. The other factor that could contribute to the variability of RELM severity may be the volumetric burden of the leaflet thrombus. It is also technically feasible to quantify the volume of the hypoattenuated region by setting a specific Hounsfield unit (HU) range for detection, although there could be considerable software limitations in this regard, because there are only a few software programs available for this purpose to the the authors' knowledge. The authors have used Mimics software (Materialise NV, Leuven, Belgium) for this purpose by setting the lower HU range of detection to −200 and the upper HU range to 200.

BIOPROSTHETIC LEAFLET ORIENTATION

The orientation of bioprosthetic leaflets relative to the native sinuses of Valsalva and commissures is critical to precise localization of HALT and RELM and thus should be accurately recorded and reported according to standardized methodology. Unlike surgically implanted bioprosthetic valves, however, the orientation, depth, and geometry of which are consistently dictated by a standardized surgical technique and thus always predictable, TAVR bioprosthetic valves may be highly variable in terms of such factors. Importantly, these factors may be associated with the initial formation of subclinical leaflet thrombosis and contribute to its progression and therefore should also be delicately and systematically analyzed and documented.

A systematic nomenclature has been developed and could be used for the precise description and surveillance of leaflet abnormalities.[10] This nomenclature has been thoroughly described previously.[10] Briefly, the rules are as follows:

- If the bioprosthetic and native leaflet commissures are well aligned, bioprosthetic leaflets of the TAVR device are designated right (R), left (L), and noncoronary (N), respectively, according to the corresponding native leaflets.

- If the native commissures bisect the bioprosthetic commissures (60° rotation), then the bioprosthetic leaflets are designated RL, LN, and NR.
- If it is a lesser degree of rotation (±30° rotation), lower-case and upper-case letters are used to designate the smaller and larger portion of the affected bioprosthetic leaflets, respectively; under such circumstances, there are 6 additional variations: Rl, Ln, Nr, rL, lN, and nR.

SUMMARY

In summary, a systematic and standardized methodology has been developed for the detection and precise assessment of leaflet thrombosis after TAVR. This methodology, if widely adopted, may contribute to the standardization of reporting and enable broader research collaboration and hence pave the way for the better future understanding and management of this relatively common yet poorly understood phenomenon.

REFERENCES

1. Mack MJ, Leon MB, Smith CR, et al. 5-year outcomes of transcatheter aortic valve replacement or surgical aortic valve replacement for high surgical risk patients with aortic stenosis (PARTNER 1): a randomised controlled trial. Lancet 2015;385(9986): 2477–84.
2. Makkar RR, Fontana G, Jilaihawi H, et al. Possible subclinical leaflet thrombosis in bioprosthetic aortic valves. N Engl J Med 2015;373(21):2015–24.
3. Pache G, Schoechlin S, Blanke P, et al. Early hypo-attenuated leaflet thickening in balloon-expandable transcatheter aortic heart valves. Eur Heart J 2016;37(28):2263–71.
4. Hansson NC, Grove EL, Andersen HR, et al. Transcatheter aortic valve thrombosis: incidence, predisposing factors, and clinical implications. J Am Coll Cardiol 2016;68(19):2059–69.
5. Chakravarty T, Søndergaard L, Friedman J, et al. Subclinical leaflet thrombosis in surgical and transcatheter bioprosthetic aortic valves: an observational study. Lancet 2017;389(10087): 2383–92.
6. Franzone A, Pilgrim T, Haynes AG, et al. Transcatheter aortic valve thrombosis: incidence, clinical presentation and long-term outcomes. Eur Heart J Cardiovasc Imaging 2018;19(4):398–404.
7. Vollema EM, Kong WKF, Katsanos S, et al. Transcatheter aortic valve thrombosis: the relation between hypo-attenuated leaflet thickening, abnormal valve haemodynamics, and stroke. Eur Heart J 2017;38(16):1207–17.
8. Sondergaard L, De Backer O, Kofoed KF, et al. Natural history of subclinical leaflet thrombosis affecting motion in bioprosthetic aortic valves. Eur Heart J 2017;38(28):2201–7.
9. Holmes DR, Mack MJ. Uncertainty and possible subclinical valve leaflet thrombosis. N Engl J Med 2015;373(21):2080–2.
10. Jilaihawi H, Asch FM, Manasse E, et al. Systematic CT methodology for the evaluation of subclinical leaflet thrombosis. JACC Cardiovasc Imaging 2017;10(4):461–70.
11. Tan N, Liu Y, Chen J-Y, et al. Use of the contrast volume or grams of iodine–to–creatinine clearance ratio to predict mortality after percutaneous coronary intervention. Am Heart J 2013;165(4): 600–8.
12. Gurm HS, Dixon SR, Smith DE, et al. Renal function-based contrast dosing to define safe limits of radiographic contrast media in patients undergoing percutaneous coronary interventions. J Am Coll Cardiol 2011;58(9):907–14.

Computed Tomography Assessment for Transcatheter Aortic Valve Replacement

Mohamad Alkhouli, MD[a],*, Lana Winkler, MD[b],
Robert J. Tallaksen, MD[b]

KEYWORDS

- Transcatheter aortic valve replacement • CT • Annular sizing • Paravalvular regurgitation
- 3-D printing • Leaflet thrombosis

KEY POINTS

- CT is the modality of choice for preprocedural assessment of vascular access, aortic annulus size, aortic arch suitability for embolic protection devices, and anticipation of coplanar fluoroscopic angulation in patients undergoing transcatheter aortic valve replacement.
- Data afforded by CT predict periprocedural complications, such as paravalvular regurgitation and annular injury. There is also emerging evidence of a potential value of CT in predicting physical recovery and long-term mortality.
- CT is playing an increasing role in postprocedural assessment of paravalvular regurgitation and subclinical leaflet thrombosis.
- Advances in computer simulation software and 3-D tissue printing technologies may expand the utility of CT to cutting-edge applications in the bioengineering and refinement of future transcatheter aortic valve therapies.

Transcatheter aortic valve replacement (TAVR) has become an important therapeutic option for patients with severe symptomatic aortic stenosis at intermediate or higher risk for surgery.[1] The introduction with TAVR has led to a surge of clinical investigations in the field of multimodality imaging due to the challenges with the design and delivery of transcatheter heart valves (THVs). In the early experience with TAVR, echocardiography was the primary imaging modality used to assess suitability for transcatheter valve intervention, to provide annular sizing and to monitor periprocedural complications, whereas the role of computed tomography (CT) was limited to access site evaluation.[2] Multidetector CT quickly gained acceptance, however, as the method of choice for pre-TAVR annular measurement due to its superior

sizing accuracy and the wealth of additional pertinent information it provides.[3,4]

This article aims to describe the role of CT in the comprehensive assessment of TAVR from the perspective of the interventional cardiologist.

TECHNICAL CONSIDERATIONS

Discussion of CT acquisition techniques and protocols is beyond the scope of this review. Technical issues with pre-TAVR CT imaging that are relevant to the interventionalists are, however, worth a brief mention.

Pre-computed Tomography Medications
Ideal acquisition protocols aim to provide a motion-free image of the aortic root as much

Disclosures: None.
[a] Division of Cardiovascular Disease, Structural Heart Interventions, West Virginia University School of Medicine, West Virginia University, 1 Medical Center Drive, Morgantown, WV 26505-8059, USA; [b] Department of Radiology, West Virginia University, 1 medical drive, Morgantown, WV 26505, USA
* Corresponding author.
E-mail address: mohamad.alkhouli@wvumedicine.org

Intervent Cardiol Clin 7 (2018) 301–313
https://doi.org/10.1016/j.iccl.2018.03.004

as possible, which heavily depends on optimal electrocardiographic gating. This requires controlling rapid heart rates and/or arrhythmias, which is usually assisted with the administration of β-blockers. However, β-blockers may not be well tolerated by the TAVR population due to the nature of aortic stenosis.[5] Similarly, unless concomitant delineation of coronary anatomy is necessary, avoidance of nitrates is preferred in these patients.

Contrast Load

Patients referred for TAVR are older and have more comorbidities and a higher incidence of renal dysfunction compared with patients who are referred for surgical aortic valve replacement. Therefore, in patients with renal dysfunction, minimizing the contrast load is paramount to avoid permanent kidney damage. This can be done by (1) lowering contrast load: reliable measurements of the aortic root can be achieved with lower contrast volumes than what are needed in coronary CT angiography; therefore, lowering the contrast volume to less than 40 mL is feasible without affecting the image quality for the purpose of TAVR in the majority of cases[5–7]; (2) staging of contrast loads: in patients with borderline renal function, limiting the CT assessment to the aortic root in one setting is desired; evaluation of the iliofemoral vasculature can then be done either by nonenhanced CT (which is usually adequate for anatomy and calcification assessment) or with direct low-volume intra-arterial contrast injection[5,7]; coronary angiography ideally should not be performed on the same day as the CT in these patients; and (3) alternative imaging with 3-D echocardiography: although CT is the method of choice for pre-TAVR assessment, contemporary 3-D transesophageal echo software has shown excellent accuracy and reproducibility of aortic root measurement in comparison with CT[8,9]; automated software can, therefore, be used in patients with advanced renal dysfunction to minimize the risk of further deterioration in renal functions.

PREPROCEDURAL PLANNING

The goals of pre-TAVR CT are to evaluate iliofemoral and alternative access routes, provide accurate sizing of the aortic annulus, determine suitability of embolic protection device (EPD) placement, anticipate fluoroscopic angles for coaxial deployment of the THV, and predict complications.

Access Evaluation

Iliofemoral access is the preferred route for THV delivery. Although modern refinements in THV delivery systems have allowed the utilization of this route in a majority of patients, alternative routes are occasionally required. These routes include transapical, direct aortic, supranotch direct aortic, subclavian, transaxillary, antegrade transseptal, and carotid and transcaval access. CT imaging is essential to assess the feasibility of iliofemoral access and is the optimal alternative access if the femoral and/or the iliac artery is heavily diseased. Issues pertaining to access suitability and imaging techniques of the vasculature are covered in a separate article in this issue.

Sizing of Transcatheter Heart Valves

The aortic annulus is a virtual ring that is defined by the lowest hinge points of the aortic valve. Inappropriate sizing (undersizing or oversizing) of THVs are associated with paravalvular regurgitation (PVR), annular rupture, device embolization, and coronary occlusion.[10,11] Therefore, accurate annular sizing is paramount to optimize TAVR outcomes. Contrary to surgically placed valves, in which the size of the valve is determined intraoperatively under direct vision using valve sizers, THVs are sized preoperatively via indirect imaging modalities. It is well established that CT allows more accurate annular sizing than 2-D echocardiography due to the ovoid or elliptical shapes of the annulus.[4] In addition, postprocessing software now allows simplified and reproducible methods of aortic annulus identification. After identifying the lowest insertion point of each of the 3 leaflets, several annular sizing parameters can be calculated (diameter, area, perimeter, and area and perimeter–derived mean diameter) (Fig. 1). Among these, the ideal parameter for annular sizing needs to integrate dimensions across the multidimensional annular plane, be stable during the cardiac cycle, and be independent of the annular shape.[5] Both the area and the perimeter fulfill these requirements to some extent, although the perimeter is less affected by noncircular annular shapes than area. In practice, area sizing is the main parameter used to determine the valve size in balloon-expandable THV implantations, whereas the perimeter is the preferred parameter used to determine the ideal self-expandable valve size. The manufacturers of the 2 commercially available devices in the United States (Sapien XT and Sapien S3 [Edwards Lifesciences, Irvine, California] and CoreValve Evolut R [Medtronic, Minneapolis, Minnesota]) provide specific sizing recommendations for their THVs

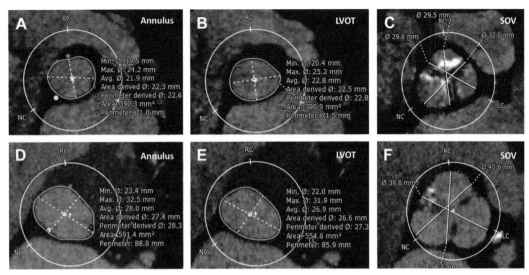

Fig. 1. Aortic annulus sizing with CT. (A–C) CT measurements of the aortic annulus, LVOT, and SOV in a patient with a small cylindrical annulus. (D–F) CT measurements of the aortic annulus, LVOT, and SOV in a patient with a large oval-shaped annulus. SOV, sinus of Valsalva.

(Table 1). For balloon-expandable valves, although only nominal balloon inflations are recommended per the instructions for use, it is not uncommon to deviate from the recommended nominal balloon inflations in several clinical scenarios: (1) in patients with borderline annulus dimensions, a strategy of THV underexpansion and ad hoc postdilation has been shown effective in achieving adequate peri-THV seal and mitigating the feared risk of annular injury with nominal balloon inflations[12,13]; (2) postdilation of the THV with supranominal balloon inflation is commonly used in with significant patient-prosthesis mismatch or moderate to severe PVR after nominal deployment; this strategy was used in 12.7% of patients in the PARTNER (The Placement of Aortic Transcatheter Valves) I trial and in 22% of patients in the CoreValve US clinical trials[14,15]; in the PARTNER 1 trial, postdilation was associated with higher rates of subacute strokes (4.9% vs 2.6%; $P = .04$), whereas in the CoreValve US trials, no excess neurologic events were observed but patients who had postdilation had higher incidence of acute kidney injury (12.7% vs 9.9%, $P<.05$)[12,14]; and (3) overexpansion of the largest THV to accommodate annuli outside of the recommended range up to (793 mm^2) has also been reported.[16]

Table 1			
Valve size selection recommendation for the commercially available valves in the United States			
Recommended Sizing for Sapien S3 Balloon-Expandable Valve			
Area	Area-Derived Diameter	Recommended Valve	Nominal Balloon Volume
273–345 mm^2	18.6–21 mm	20 mm	11 mL
338–430 mm^2	20.7–23.4 mm	23 mm	17 mL
430–546 mm^2	23.4–26.4 mm	26 mm	23 mL
540–683 mm^2	26.2–29.5 mm	29 mm	33 mL
Recommended Sizing for Evolut R Self-Expandable Valve			
Perimeter	Perimeter-Derived Diameter	Recommended Valve	Postdilation Balloon
56.2–62.8 mm	18–20 mm	23 mm	22 mm
62.8–72.3 mm	20–23 mm	26 mm	25 mm
72.3–81.7 mm	23–26 mm	29 mm	28 mm
81.7–94.2 mm	26–30 mm	34 mm	30 mm

Implantation Angle Prediction

Coaxial device implantation is essential to the optimization of TAVR outcomes. Malpositioning of THV is associated with several potential complications (PVR, device embolization, need for pacemaker, and so forth).[10] CT affords 3-D orientation of the annular plane, from which a line of perpendicularity can be obtained.[17] This line provides an infinite number of angles that are perpendicular to the valve plane in a given patient; any of these angles can be used at the time of THV implantation.[5,17] Once a specific angle is selected, aortic root angiography is usually performed to confirm perpendicularity. In an average patient, the line of perpendicularity runs from a right anterior oblique-caudal projection, crosses the posterior-anterior projection at approximately 10° caudal and the straight left anterior oblique at approximately 10° and then continues with increasing cranial requirements for steeper left anterior oblique projections.[5] Steep and unusual projections, however, might be necessary in patients with kyphoscoliosis or horizontal or unfolded aortas. This is particularly important because it may have implications on THV selection, because increased aortic root angulations have been found to attenuate procedural success after self-expandable but not balloon-expandable TAVR.[18] Angle prediction can also be achieved with good accuracy using 3-D angiographic reconstructions.[19] CT coplanar angle prediction, however, enjoys higher reproducibility and does not require additional contrast. It does, nonetheless, have a learning curve and require high-quality data acquisition and good patient positioning.[5]

Determining Suitability of Cerebral Embolic Protection Devices

Cerebral EPDs have gained substantial interest recently due to their potential role in reducing debris embolization to the brain during TAVR. The Sentinel System (Claret Medical, Santa Rosa, California) is the first device approved by the Food and Drug Administration for routine use during TAVR.[20,21] Typically advanced via the right radial or brachial artery, the Sentinel System is composed of 2 filters: a proximal filter that is placed in the aortic arch takeoff section of the brachiocephalic artery and a distal filter that is placed in the proximal part of the left common carotid artery. CT provides a wealth of data on the aortic arch anatomy, which allows the operator to determine feasibility of EPDs and increase the safety of their use. Severe tortuosity of the right innominate artery, heavy calcifications of the arch vessels, and some anatomic variation of the aortic arch increase procedural complexity and may limit an operator's ability to deploy the filters and possibly increase the risk of complications (**Fig. 2**). Another relevant potential utility of the pre-TAVR CT is to predict stroke risk based on the burden of aortic valve plaque/calcifications. In a study of 91 patients undergoing TAVR with Sapien XT THVs, preprocedural CT measurement of the volume of aortic valve plaque was predictive of ischemic stroke and neurocognitive decline.[22]

Prediction of Complications
Annular rupture

The presence of landing zone calcification is key to adequately anchor THVs. Severe or extreme calcifications in the annulus, left ventricular outflow tract (LVOT), or the ascending aorta, however, increase the risk of procedural complications. Patients with extremely calcified aortic valves/annuli have lower device success rates with both self-expandable and balloon-expandable THVs and greater risk of PVR.[23–29] Nodular and asymmetric calcifications may increase the need for postdilation and also risk aortic perforation during balloon-expandable THV implantation (**Fig. 3**).[24,27] In these patients, self-expandable valve might be a safer alternative. Calcifications extending into the LVOT also increase the risk of both PVR and annular disruption.[30] In a study of 31 patients who suffered annular or subannular rupture, the presence of moderate to severe LVOT calcifications was the strongest predictor of this complication (odd ratio 10.92; 95% CI, 3.23–36.91; $P<.001$).[30] The presence of extreme ascending aortic calcifications has important implications for procedural planning and patients' informed decisions. Those patients need to be informed about the issues pertaining to cross-clamping of the aorta in case an open surgical bail-out is needed. Hence, quantification of the calcium burden in the LVOT, annulus, and ascending aorta is key and can often lead to important modifications in the procedural planning.

Coronary occlusion

Obstruction of the left main or the right coronary artery is a rare but potentially life-threatening complication of TAVR. This is usually due to displacement of 1 or more calcified native leaflets during valve deployment and less commonly to coverage of the coronary ostium by the valve frame or sealing cuff.[3] Migration of calcium and atheromatous plaque to the coronary bed at the time of THV implantation has also been reported.[31] In a multicenter registry, coronary

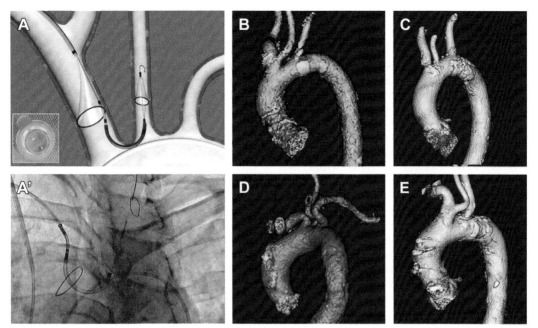

Fig. 2. Role of CT in assessing suitability of EPDs. (*A*) Illustration of the Sentinel EPD. Retrieved debris (3 mm in size) from patient after TAVR are shown in the inset. (*A'*) Fluoroscopic illustration of the placement of the Sentinel System in the left common carotid artery and the right innominate artery. VR 3-D images of the aortic arch in patients with aortic stenosis referred for TAVR. (*B*) Mildly tortuous innominate artery and a bovine arch. (*C*) Nontortuous innominate artery with normal arch. (*D*) Extremely tortuous innominate, left carotid, and left subclavian arteries. (*E*) Mildly tortuous innominate and left carotid arteries and a bovine arch.

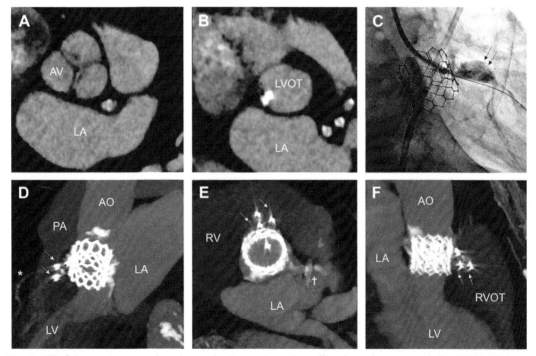

Fig. 3. CT of the aortic root and aortic annulus in a patient who suffered annular rupture during TAVR. (*A*) Aortic annulus pre-TAVR. (*B*) LVOT pre-TAVR. (*C*) Fluoroscopic illustration of the annular rupture after TAVR. (*D–F*) MPR images of the aortic annular and aortic root after percutaneous treatment of the annular injury. Red arrows, calcified nodule in the LOVT just below the noncoronary and the left coronary cusp; black arrows, site of annular perforation with bleeding into the pericardium; yellow arrows, Amplatzer (St Jude Medical, Minneapolis, MN) ductal occluders sealing the perforation; asterisk, right coronary artery; cross, left main coronary artery. AV, aortic valve; LA, left atrium; LV, left ventricle; PA, pulmonary artery; RV, right ventricle; RVOT, right ventricular outflow tract. (*Adapted from* Alkhouli M, Carpenter E, Tarabishy A, et al. Annular rupture during transcatheter aortic valve replacement: novel treatment with amplatzer vascular plugs. Eur Heart J 2017;39(8):714–5; with permission.)

occlusion occurred in 44 of 6688 patients (0.66%) undergoing TAVR, and the left main coronary artery was involved in 88.6% of cases. Coronary height and sinus of Valsalva diameter were the most predictive anatomic factors of coronary occlusion; patients who experienced coronary occlusion had lower left coronary ostial height and sinus of Valsalva diameter (10.6 mm ± 2.1 mm vs 13.4 mm ± 2.1 mm, P<.001; 28.1 ± 3.8 mm vs 31.9 ± 4.1 mm, P<.001) compared with those who did not experience coronary occlusion. Therefore, precise measurements of the coronary ostial height and the diameter of the sinus of Valsalva and sinotubular junction are essential to avoid coronary occlusion. It is generally accepted that patients with coronary distance less than 10 mm from the annulus and those with narrow sinus of Valsalva less than 28 mm are at high risk of coronary occlusion.[32,33] In addition, the length and the bulk of calcifications of the native leaflets should be considered, because coronary occlusion has been reported despite adequate coronary height in cases where the aortic valve leaflets are long in relation to the coronary sinus dimension.[34]

Special considerations should be given to patients undergoing aortic valve-in-valve (VinV) implantation for 2 reasons: (1) VinV procedures are associated with 4-fold to 6-fold higher risk of coronary occlusion compared with TAVR[35] and (2) methods of identifying anatomic landmarks on CT in the presence of a surgical bioprothesis differ from those in patients undergoing TAVR.[36] In contrast to TAVR, coronary ostial height is less relevant in VinV implantation procedures. Rather, the proximity of the coronary ostia to the anticipated final position of the displaced bioprosthetic leaflets is the major determinant of coronary occlusion risk. This is often dictated by the existing angulation of the surgical bioprostheses because they are commonly tilted. An important term in predicting coronary occlusion with VinV is, therefore, the *virtual THV to coronary distance*, defined as the anticipated distance of the implanted THV inside the surgical bioprothesis to the coronary ostia (Fig. 4).[36] A systematic approach to estimating the risk of coronary occlusion in patients undergoing VinV implantation has been suggested by Blanke and colleagues.[36] In this algorithm, patients with stentless surgical prostheses undergo

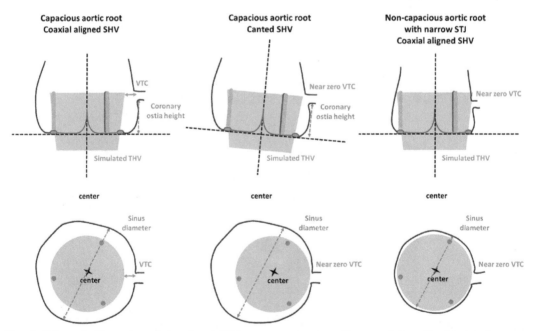

Fig. 4. Schematic illustration of the virtual THV to coronary artery distance. Schematic drawing (*top row*, long axis view; *bottom row*, short axis view) illustrating THV implantation in a stented bioprosthesis with 3 posts in 3 different scenarios: right column, coaxial aligned bioprosthesis in a capacious aortic root; middle column, a tilted bioprosthesis in a capacious aortic root; and left column, coaxial aligned bioprosthesis in a non-capacious aortic root with a narrow sinotubular junction. SHV, stented heart valve; STJ, the sinotubular junction; VTC, virtual THV to coronary distance. (*From* Blanke P, Soon J, Dvir D, et al. Computed tomography assessment for transcatheter aortic valve in valve implantation: the vancouver approach to predict anatomical risk for coronary obstruction and other considerations. J Cardiovasc Comput Tomogr 2016;10(6):491–9; with permission.)

a similar evaluation to those submitted for TAVR due to the lack of a rigid scaffold. In patients with stented surgical prostheses, however, assessment of the virtual THV to coronary distance is necessary. This is measured simply by overlying a cylinder representing the expanded THV on the middle of the basal ring using any multiplanar reformatting capable platform. This measurement can be useful in predicting coronary occlusion if the level of the coronary ostium is above the stent posts. In patients who are deemed at high risk for coronary occlusion during TAVR or VinV, preemptive coronary protection techniques (eg, guide wires and an undeployed balloon or stent in left main or right coronary artery) can be used successfully to mitigate catastrophic consequences of acute coronary occlusion.[33]

Other procedural complications

In patients with aortic stenosis and an associated asymmetrical septal hypertrophy, acute hemodynamic can occur after TAVR due to dynamic LVOT gradients after valvular afterload removal.[37,38] In these settings, CT allows prediction of this potential complication and can delineate septal anatomy for bail out alcohol septal ablation.[39,40] Pre-TAVR CT may also be able to identify anatomic predictors of the need for permanent pacemaker after TAVR. Shorter membranous septum length, larger prosthesis to LVOT ratio and prosthesis to sinus of Valsalva ratio have been shown independent predictors of permanent pacemaker need regardless of baseline conduction abnormalities.[41–43]

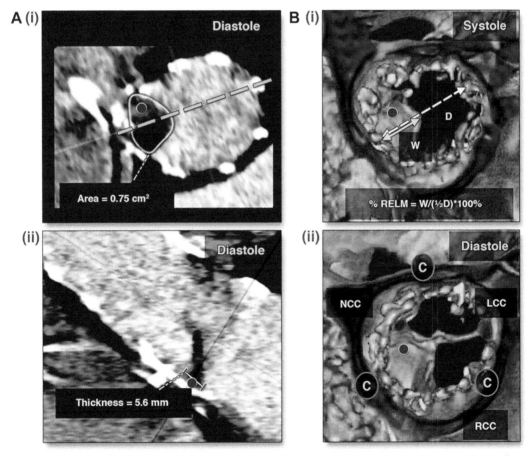

Fig. 5. Appearance of leaflet thrombosis on CT. (A) Characteristic wedge-shaped or semilunar opacities in hypo-attenuated leaflet thickening (Ai) 2-D axial MPR and (Aii) the corresponding 2-D longitudinal MPR (derived from *green dashed line* [Ai]). Additional measurement of the area and thickens of areas affected can be performed to quantify HALT. (B) Characteristic RELM seen with leaflet thrombosis. 3-D en face VR projection in both systole (Bi) (maximal leaflet opening) and diastole (Bii). A formula to quantify RELM is also illustrated (Bii). C, coplanar level; D, diameter; LCC, left coronary cusp; NCC, non coronary cusp; RCC, right coronary cusp; W, width. (*From* Jilaihawi H, Asch FM, Manasse E, et al. Systematic CT methodology for the evaluation of subclinical leaflet thrombosis. JACC Cardiovasc Imaging 2017;10(4):461–70; with permission.)

POSTPROCEDURAL ASSESSMENT

CT is not routinely performed after TAVR. Its utility has been increasingly recognized, however, in the early detection of possible post-implantation complications and in the assessment of corrective interventions of these complications.[44]

Leaflet Abnormalities

The phenomenon of early leaflet thrombosis after surgical and TAVR has recently gained substantial interest due to its potential impact on clinical outcomes.[45–47] Clinical leaflet thrombosis is uncommon and is usually considered when new echocardiographic findings of valve dysfunction are observed (mean transvalvular gradient > 20 mm Hg > mild transvalvular regurgitation) and when partial or complete resolution of these abnormalities occurs with anticoagulation.[48] Subclinical leaflet thrombosis is common, however, but its diagnosis requires a high-quality CT.[49] The hallmark CT finding of subclinical leaflet thrombosis is a combination of hypoattenuated leaflet thickening (HALT) and reduced leaflet motion (RELM).[49–51] Although HALT is assessed using a cross-sectional 2-D multiplanar reconstruction (MPR), assessing RELM requires an en face 4-D volume rendering (VR) (**Fig. 5**). An algorithmic approach to assessing leaflet abnormalities on post-TAVR CT has been suggested by Jilaihawi and colleagues.[49] Briefly, acquisition techniques should be optimized to ensure the highest possible quality CT data set. This includes full retrospective gating, utilization of a high-resolution scanner, avoidance of dose modulation, and possibly increasing the scanner acquisition voltage to 140 kV. The scan is then assessed for its technical quality per the empiric criteria suggested by Jilaihawi and colleagues; adequate scans should allow visualization of HALT on 2-D MPR and of leaflet motion through most systolic phases on 4-D VR imaging. If complete coaptation is seen on 2-D MPR, then subclinical leaflet thrombosis is ruled out. If HALT is clearly seen, then further assessment of leaflet excursion with 4-D VR is necessary; RELM is considered present when maximal leaflet opening is reduced by greater than 50%. These recommendations, however, are based on limited data. Nevertheless, several investigations are ongoing and their awaited results will aid in validating and standardizing reporting of leaflet abnormalities after bioprothestic valve replacement.

Paravalvular Regurgitation

Incidence of PVR post-TAVR has declined significantly with contemporary THVs.[1] Yet, PVR remains the Achilles heel of TAVR due to the significant morbidity and mortality associated with it.[52] In selected patients with moderate to severe PVR after TAVR, percutaneous repair is feasible and effective but is often technically challenging.[53,54] CT can facilitate identification and accurate measurement of the defect, assessment of the distance to the adjacent coronary ostium, and prediction of the optimal fluoroscopic angles to cross the defect (**Fig. 6**).[55] Acquisition protocols are similar to standard pre-TAVR protocols.

NOVEL APPLICATIONS AND FUTURE DIRECTIONS

The advances in the TAVR field brought forth an unprecedented scientific interest in cardiac CT. Novel applications of the pre-TAVR CT have been recently proposed. These include (1) developing CT-based risk prediction models to predict clinical outcomes beyond procedural complications and (2) investigating the role of computer-based simulation techniques and CT-based 3-D tissue printing in future TAVR.

Prediction of Non–valve-Related Clinical Outcomes

CT offers an abundance of raw data, some of which can serve as a surrogate to a patient's cardiovascular and overall health with potential prognostic implications. For example, fat mass and skeletal muscle mass as assessed on pre-TAVR CT have been found strong predictors of hospital length of stay and long-term mortality a TAVR.[56,57] Similarly, the ratio of aortic root area to ascending aortic height was found to improve risk stratification of cardiovascular and all-cause long-term mortality in patients with bicuspid and tricuspid aortic valve undergoing TAVR.[58,59] Pre-TAVR CT permits evaluation of not only aortic valve/root calcifications but also calcification in the mitral valve apparatus. Paucity of mitral annular calcifications and lower mitral annular diameter on pre-TAVR CT have been associated with significant improvement of mitral regurgitation after TAVR.[60]

Computer-Based Simulation and 3-D Tissue Printing

Using finite elements analysis of the aortic valve/root and the adjacent structures,

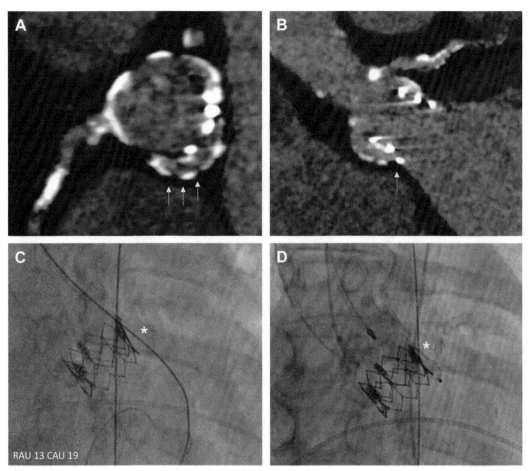

Fig. 6. CT assessment in a patient with severe PVR after TAVR. (*A, B*) Cross-sectional views illustrating a large communication between the left ventricle and the aorta outside of the transcatheter valve (*yellow arrows*). (*C, D*) Fluoroscopic illustration of crossing of the leak and percutaneous closure (*asterisks*).

computational models can be reconstructed from the pre-TAVR multislice CT to simulate THV deployment. This allows prediction of stress distributions, geometric changes, coaptation values, and risk of PVR after TAVR.[61] Recent studies have shown an incremental value to printing graspable 3-D models for periprocedural planning of TAVR[62]; Qian and colleagues[63] demonstrated the feasibility of using 3-D printed tissue-mimicking phantoms to quantitatively assess post-TAVR aortic root strain and strain unevenness in vitro (**Fig. 7**). These parameters achieved high accuracy value in predicting post-TAVR PVR. Maragiannis and colleagues[64] successfully applied 3-D printing technologies to develop patient-specific models of the anatomic and functional characteristics of severe aortic stenosis. These patient-specific models, albeit new and requiring further validation, can be used to predict and improve the acute hemodynamic performance of THV treatment strategies and to refine quantification methods of aortic stenosis in certain challenging subgroups of patients (eg, low flow and low gradient). Another appealing feature of 3-D printed models is their potential ability to test, improve, or design new THVs.[65] Computer simulation and 3-D printing techniques, however, must first be standardized, validated, and made cost-effective before their application becomes mainstream in the field of TAVR.[66] Nonetheless, a central role for these novel technologies in the future of transcatheter aortic valve therapies can be speculated. Perhaps both modalities can be integrated where personalized tissue valves can be optimized pioneered and assessed with computer simulation analyses and then 3-D printed and further refined in vitro to achieve the ideal valve model.[52]

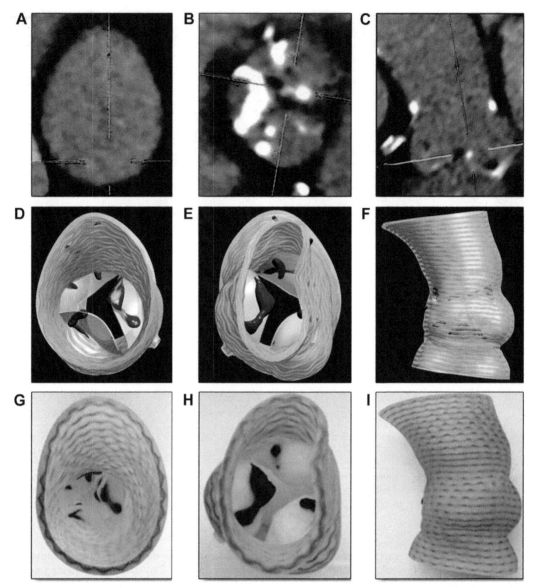

Fig. 7. CT cross-sectional views with a derived 3-D printed phantoms of the aortic annulus and aortic root in a patient with aortic stenosis. (*A–C*) Cross-sectional views of aortic annulus and the ascending aorta. (*D–F*) 3-D computational models showing the ascending aorta (*D*), the LVOT (*E*), and the side (*F*). Calcifications are drawn in red. The embedded fibers were drawn in green. (*G–I*) A 3-D printed phantom of the aortic annulus and the aortic root. The calcifications and the fibers were printed with black materials for better illustration. (*From* Qian Z, Wang K, Liu S, et al. Quantitative prediction of paravalvular leak in transcatheter aortic valve replacement based on tissue-mimicking 3D printing. JACC Cardiovasc Imaging 2017;10(7):719–31; with permission.)

SUMMARY

CT has become as essential element of modern TAVR, with an established utility in vascular access evaluation, aortic annular measurement, and prediction of periprocedural complications. Nevertheless, with the underrepresented advances in imaging technology, a more pivotal role for CT can be foreseen in the innovation and application of future THV therapies.

REFERENCES

1. Vahl TP, Kodali SK, Leon MB. Transcatheter aortic valve replacement 2016: a modern-day "through the looking-glass" adventure. J Am Coll Cardiol 2016;67(12):1472–87.
2. Anwaruddin S. The role of preoperative and intraoperative imaging in guiding transcatheter aortic valve replacement. Interv Cardiol Clin 2015;4(1): 39–51.

3. Leipsic J, Yang TH, Min JK. Computed tomographic imaging of transcatheter aortic valve replacement for prediction and prevention of procedural complications. Circ Cardiovasc Imaging 2013;6(4):597–605.

4. Jilaihawi H, Kashif M, Fontana G, et al. Cross-sectional computed tomographic assessment improves accuracy of aortic annular sizing for transcatheter aortic valve replacement and reduces the incidence of paravalvular aortic regurgitation. J Am Coll Cardiol 2012;59(14):1275–86.

5. Apfaltrer P, Henzler T, Blanke P, et al. Computed tomography for planning transcatheter aortic valve replacement. J Thorac Imaging 2013;28(4):231–9.

6. Felmly LM, De Cecco CN, Schoepf UJ, et al. Low contrast medium-volume third-generation dual-source computed tomography angiography for transcatheter aortic valve replacement planning. Eur Radiol 2017;27(5):1944–53.

7. Khalique OK, Pulerwitz TC, Halliburton SS, et al. Practical considerations for optimizing cardiac computed tomography protocols for comprehensive acquisition prior to transcatheter aortic valve replacement. J Cardiovasc Comput Tomogr 2016; 10(5):364–74.

8. Prihadi EA, van Rosendael PJ, Vollema EM, et al. Feasibility, accuracy, and reproducibility of aortic annular and root sizing for transcatheter aortic valve replacement using novel automated three-dimensional echocardiographic software: comparison with multi-detector row computed tomography. J Am Soc Echocardiogr 2018;31(4):505–14.e3.

9. Jilaihawi H, Doctor N, Kashif M, et al. Aortic annular sizing for transcatheter aortic valve replacement using cross-sectional 3-dimensional transesophageal echocardiography. J Am Coll Cardiol 2013;61(9):908–16.

10. Binder RK, Webb JG, Willson AB, et al. The impact of integration of a multidetector computed tomography annulus area sizing algorithm on outcomes of transcatheter aortic valve replacement: a prospective, multicenter, controlled trial. J Am Coll Cardiol 2013;62(5):431–8.

11. Yang TH, Webb JG, Blanke P, et al. Incidence and severity of paravalvular aortic regurgitation with multidetector computed tomography nominal area oversizing or undersizing after transcatheter heart valve replacement with the Sapien 3: a comparison with the Sapien XT. JACC Cardiovasc Interv 2015;8(3):462–71.

12. Barbanti M, Leipsic J, Binder R, et al. Underexpansion and ad hoc post-dilation in selected patients undergoing balloon-expandable transcatheter aortic valve replacement. J Am Coll Cardiol 2014; 63(10):976–81.

13. Tan JS, Leipsic J, Perlman G, et al. A Strategy of underexpansion and ad hoc post-dilation of balloon-expandable transcatheter aortic valves in patients at risk of annular injury: favorable mid-term outcomes. JACC Cardiovasc Interv 2015; 8(13):1727–32.

14. Harrison JK, Hughes GC, Reardon MJ, et al. Balloon post-dilation following implantation of a self-expanding transcatheter aortic valve bioprosthesis. JACC Cardiovasc Interv 2017;10(2):168–75.

15. Hahn RT, Pibarot P, Webb J, et al. Outcomes with post-dilation following transcatheter aortic valve replacement: the PARTNER I trial (placement of aortic transcatheter valve). JACC Cardiovasc Interv 2014;7(7):781–9.

16. Mathur M, McCabe JM, Aldea G, et al. Overexpansion of the 29 mm SAPIEN 3 transcatheter heart valve in patients with large aortic annuli (area > 683 mm(2)): a case series. Catheter Cardiovasc Interv 2017. [Epub ahead of print].

17. Gurvitch R, Wood DA, Leipsic J, et al. Multislice computed tomography for prediction of optimal angiographic deployment projections during transcatheter aortic valve implantation. JACC Cardiovasc Interv 2010;3(11):1157–65.

18. Abramowitz Y, Maeno Y, Chakravarty T, et al. Aortic angulation attenuates procedural success following self-expandable but not balloon-expandable TAVR. JACC Cardiovasc Imaging 2016;9(8):964–72.

19. Binder RK, Leipsic J, Wood D, et al. Prediction of optimal deployment projection for transcatheter aortic valve replacement: angiographic 3-dimensional reconstruction of the aortic root versus multidetector computed tomography. Circ Cardiovasc Interv 2012;5(2):247–52.

20. Kapadia SR, Kodali S, Makkar R, et al. Protection against cerebral embolism during transcatheter aortic valve replacement. J Am Coll Cardiol 2017; 69(4):367–77.

21. Seeger J, Gonska B, Otto M, et al. Cerebral embolic protection during transcatheter aortic valve replacement significantly reduces death and stroke compared with unprotected procedures. JACC Cardiovasc Interv 2017;10(22):2297–303.

22. Tada N, Haga Y, Suzuki S, et al. Computed tomography score of aortic valve tissue may predict cerebral embolism during transcatheter aortic valve implantation. JACC Cardiovasc Imaging 2017; 10(8):960–2.

23. Abramowitz Y, Jilaihawi H, Chakravarty T, et al. Balloon-expandable transcatheter aortic valve replacement in patients with extreme aortic valve calcification. Catheter Cardiovasc Interv 2016; 87(6):1173–9.

24. Khalique OK, Hahn RT, Gada H, et al. Quantity and location of aortic valve complex calcification predicts severity and location of paravalvular regurgitation

and frequency of post-dilation after balloon-expandable transcatheter aortic valve replacement. JACC Cardiovasc Interv 2014;7(8):885–94.

25. Stahli BE, Nguyen-Kim TD, Gebhard C, et al. Prosthesis-specific predictors of paravalvular regurgitation after transcatheter aortic valve replacement: impact of calcification and sizing on balloon-expandable versus self-expandable transcatheter heart valves. J Heart Valve Dis 2015;24(1):10–21.

26. Azzalini L, Ghoshhajra BB, Elmariah S, et al. The aortic valve calcium nodule score (AVCNS) independently predicts paravalvular regurgitation after transcatheter aortic valve replacement (TAVR). J Cardiovasc Comput Tomogr 2014;8(2):131–40.

27. Alkhouli M, Carpenter E, Tarabishy A, et al. Annular rupture during transcatheter aortic valve replacement: novel treatment with amplatzer vascular plugs. Eur Heart J 2017;39(8):714–5.

28. Pasic M, Unbehaun A, Buz S, et al. Annular rupture during transcatheter aortic valve replacement: classification, pathophysiology, diagnostics, treatment approaches, and prevention. JACC Cardiovasc Interv 2015;8(1 Pt A):1–9.

29. Hansson NC, Norgaard BL, Barbanti M, et al. The impact of calcium volume and distribution in aortic root injury related to balloon-expandable transcatheter aortic valve replacement. J Cardiovasc Comput Tomogr 2015;9(5):382–92.

30. Barbanti M, Yang TH, Rodes Cabau J, et al. Anatomical and procedural features associated with aortic root rupture during balloon-expandable transcatheter aortic valve replacement. Circulation 2013;128(3):244–53.

31. Hong SJ, Hong MK, Ko YG, et al. Migration of calcium and atheromatous plaque in computed tomography: an important mechanism of coronary artery occlusion after transcatheter aortic valve replacement. J Am Coll Cardiol 2014;63(12):e23.

32. Akinseye OA, Jha SK, Ibebuogu UN. Clinical outcomes of coronary occlusion following transcatheter aortic valve replacement: a systematic review. Cardiovasc Revasc Med 2017. [Epub ahead of print].

33. Abramowitz Y, Chakravarty T, Jilaihawi H, et al. Clinical impact of coronary protection during transcatheter aortic valve implantation: first reported series of patients. EuroIntervention 2015;11(5):572–81.

34. Okuyama K, Jilaihawi H, Makkar RR. Leaflet length and left main coronary artery occlusion following transcatheter aortic valve replacement. Catheter Cardiovasc Interv 2013;82(5):E754–9.

35. Dvir D, Leipsic J, Blanke P, et al. Coronary obstruction in transcatheter aortic valve-in-valve implantation: preprocedural evaluation, device selection, protection, and treatment. Circ Cardiovasc Interv 2015;8(1) [pii:e002079].

36. Blanke P, Soon J, Dvir D, et al. Computed tomography assessment for transcatheter aortic valve in valve implantation: the vancouver approach to predict anatomical risk for coronary obstruction and other considerations. J Cardiovasc Comput Tomogr 2016;10(6):491–9.

37. Sorajja P, Booker JD, Rihal CS. Alcohol septal ablation after transaortic valve implantation: the dynamic nature of left outflow tract obstruction. Catheter Cardiovasc Interv 2013;81(2):387–91.

38. Suh WM, Witzke CF, Palacios IF. Suicide left ventricle following transcatheter aortic valve implantation. Catheter Cardiovasc Interv 2010;76(4):616–20.

39. Yanagiuchi T, Tada N, Mizutani Y, et al. Feasibility assessment of alcohol septal ablation in transcatheter aortic valve replacement using multidetector computed tomography. JACC Cardiovasc Interv 2017;10(2):e7–9.

40. Sayah N, Urena M, Brochet E, et al. Alcohol septal ablation preceding transcatheter valve implantation to prevent left ventricular outflow tract obstruction. EuroIntervention 2017. [Epub ahead of print].

41. Maeno Y, Abramowitz Y, Kawamori H, et al. A highly predictive risk model for pacemaker implantation after TAVR. JACC Cardiovasc Imaging 2017;10(10 Pt A):1139–47.

42. Routh JM, Joseph L, Marthaler BR, et al. Imaging-based predictors of permanent pacemaker implantation after transcatheter aortic valve replacement. Pacing Clin Electrophysiol 2017;41(1):81–6.

43. Nazif TM, Dizon JM, Hahn RT, et al. Predictors and clinical outcomes of permanent pacemaker implantation after transcatheter aortic valve replacement: the PARTNER (Placement of AoRtic TraNscathetER Valves) trial and registry. JACC Cardiovasc Interv 2015;8(1 Pt A):60–9.

44. Al-Najafi S, Sanchez F, Lerakis S. The crucial role of cardiac imaging in transcatheter aortic valve replacement (TAVR): pre- and post-procedural assessment. Curr Treat Options Cardiovasc Med 2016;18(12):70.

45. Jose J, Sulimov DS, El-Mawardy M, et al. Clinical bioprosthetic heart valve thrombosis after transcatheter aortic valve replacement: incidence, characteristics, and treatment outcomes. JACC Cardiovasc Interv 2017;10(7):686–97.

46. Makkar RR, Fontana G, Jilaihawi H, et al. Possible subclinical leaflet thrombosis in bioprosthetic aortic valves. N Engl J Med 2015;373(21):2015–24.

47. Chakravarty T, Sondergaard L, Friedman J, et al. Subclinical leaflet thrombosis in surgical and transcatheter bioprosthetic aortic valves: an observational study. Lancet 2017;389(10087):2383–92.

48. Latib A, Naganuma T, Abdel-Wahab M, et al. Treatment and clinical outcomes of transcatheter heart valve thrombosis. Circ Cardiovasc Interv 2015;8(4) [pii:e001779].

49. Jilaihawi H, Asch FM, Manasse E, et al. Systematic CT methodology for the evaluation of subclinical

leaflet thrombosis. JACC Cardiovasc Imaging 2017; 10(4):461–70.

50. Pache G, Schoechlin S, Blanke P, et al. Early hypoattenuated leaflet thickening in balloon-expandable transcatheter aortic heart valves. Eur Heart J 2016; 37(28):2263–71.

51. Marwan M, Mekkhala N, Goller M, et al. Leaflet thrombosis following transcatheter aortic valve implantation. J Cardiovasc Comput Tomogr 2017; 12(1):8–13.

52. Alkhouli M, Sengupta PP. 3-Dimensional-printed models for TAVR planning: why guess when you can see? JACC Cardiovasc Imaging 2017;10(7):732–4.

53. Waterbury TM, Reeder GS, Pislaru SV, et al. Techniques and outcomes of paravalvular leak repair after transcatheter aortic valve replacement. Catheter Cardiovasc Interv 2017;90(5):870–7.

54. Dhoble A, Chakravarty T, Nakamura M, et al. Outcome of paravalvular leak repair after transcatheter aortic valve replacement with a balloon-expandable prosthesis. Catheter Cardiovasc Interv 2017;89(3):462–8.

55. Alkhouli M, Sarraf M, Maor E, et al. Techniques and outcomes of percutaneous aortic paravalvular leak closure. JACC Cardiovasc Interv 2016;9(23):2416–26.

56. Dahya V, Xiao J, Prado CM, et al. Computed tomography-derived skeletal muscle index: a novel predictor of frailty and hospital length of stay after transcatheter aortic valve replacement. Am Heart J 2016;182:21–7.

57. Mok M, Allende R, Leipsic J, et al. Prognostic value of fat mass and skeletal muscle mass determined by computed tomography in patients who underwent transcatheter aortic valve implantation. Am J Cardiol 2016;117(5):828–33.

58. Masri A, Kalahasti V, Svensson LG, et al. Aortic cross-sectional area/height ratio and outcomes in patients with bicuspid aortic valve and a dilated ascending aorta. Circ Cardiovasc Imaging 2017; 10(6):e006249.

59. Masri A, Kalahasti V, Svensson LG, et al. Aortic cross-sectional area/height ratio and outcomes in patients with a trileaflet aortic valve and a dilated aorta. Circulation 2016;134(22):1724–37.

60. Amat-Santos IJ, Revilla A, Lopez J, et al. Value of CT in patients undergoing self-expandable TAVR to assess outcomes of concomitant mitral regurgitation. JACC Cardiovasc Imaging 2015;8(2):226–7.

61. Wang Q, Primiano C, McKay R, et al. CT image-based engineering analysis of transcatheter aortic valve replacement. JACC Cardiovasc Imaging 2014;7(5):526–8.

62. Ripley B, Kelil T, Cheezum MK, et al. 3D printing based on cardiac CT assists anatomic visualization prior to transcatheter aortic valve replacement. J Cardiovasc Comput Tomogr 2016;10(1):28–36.

63. Qian Z, Wang K, Liu S, et al. Quantitative prediction of paravalvular leak in transcatheter aortic valve replacement based on tissue-mimicking 3D printing. JACC Cardiovasc Imaging 2017;10(7):719–31.

64. Maragiannis D, Jackson MS, Igo SR, et al. Replicating patient-specific severe aortic valve stenosis with functional 3D modeling. Circ Cardiovasc Imaging 2015;8(10):e003626.

65. Vukicevic M, Mosadegh B, Min JK, et al. Cardiac 3D printing and its future directions. JACC Cardiovasc Imaging 2017;10(2):171–84.

66. Mathur M, Patil P, Bove A. The role of 3D printing in Structural heart disease: all that glitters is not gold. JACC Cardiovasc Imaging 2015;8(8):987–8.

Intravascular Ultrasound for Guidance and Optimization of Percutaneous Coronary Intervention

Dhruv Mahtta, MD, MBA[a], Akram Y. Elgendy, MD[b],
Islam Y. Elgendy, MD, FESC[b], Ahmed N. Mahmoud, MD[b],
Jonathan M. Tobis, MD, MSCAI[c],
Mohammad K. Mojadidi, MD[b],*

KEYWORDS

- Intravascular ultrasound • Percutaneous coronary intervention • Drug-eluting stent
- Major adverse cardiac events • Minimum lumen diameter • Minimum lumen area • Planimetry

---

KEY POINTS

- Conventional angiography provides a 2-dimensional silhouette that delivers a suboptimal assessment of true physiologic coronary artery stenosis.
- Intravascular ultrasound allows visualization of the trilaminar coronary vasculature, permitting better delineation of the quantity and quality of plaque burden.
- Clinical outcomes with intravascular ultrasound-guided interventions have revealed improved results, especially for complex and long coronary artery lesions.
- Parameters measured by intravascular ultrasound show modest correlation with other investigatory modalities.
- The use of intravascular ultrasound during routine percutaneous coronary intervention is not widely adopted, which may be in part due to equipment costs and increased procedural times.

BACKGROUND

Coronary angiography with percutaneous coronary intervention (PCI) is considered the reference standard for management of symptomatic stable coronary artery disease refractory to optimal medical management, and acute coronary syndromes.[1,2] Although conventional angiography has been used as the predominant technique to define the coronary anatomy and guide PCI, several shortcomings of this modality hinder achieving optimal results. Questions about the accuracy of coronary angiography dates to the 1970s, when researchers investigated discrepancies between a coronary lesion's appearance on angiography compared with its true physiologic effects on the myocardium.[3,4] Conventional angiography is limited by a 2-dimensional projection of the arterial lumen as well as complexity of coronary lesions, such as tortuosity or overlap of structures.[5,6] Studies have shown that there is a large degree of

---

Disclosure Statement: Dr J.M. Tobis was a consultant for St. Jude Medical Inc and W.L. Gore and Associates. All other authors report no conflict of interest.
[a] Department of Medicine, University of Florida, 1600 Southwest Archer Road, Gainesville, FL 32610, USA;
[b] Division of Cardiovascular Medicine, Department of Medicine, University of Florida, 1600 Southwest Archer Road, Gainesville, FL 32610, USA; [c] Program in Interventional Cardiology, Division of Cardiology, University of California, Los Angeles, 10833 Le Conte Avenue, Factor Building CHS, Room B-976, Los Angeles, CA 90095, USA
* Corresponding author. Division of Cardiovascular Medicine, University of Florida, 1600 Southwest Archer Road, Gainesville, FL 32610.
E-mail address: mkmojadidi@gmail.com

interobserver and intraobserver variability in assessing the degree of coronary stenosis.[7–9] The conventional methodology of quantifying stenotic lesions via their angiographic appearance relies heavily on the surrounding "nondiseased" lumen, which serves as the reference segment. However, because of diffuse involvement of the atherosclerotic disease process, a reference "nondiseased" segment is often unavailable.[10,11] The 2-dimensional planar silhouette during angiography in conjunction with a diffuse and symmetrically diseased artery poses a challenge for true physiologic assessment of a stenotic coronary lesion. Furthermore, this suboptimal visualization of stenotic lesions is compounded when PCI is performed under angiographic guidance. Conventional angiographic guidance may prohibit accurate deployment of balloons and sizing of stents, which may result in downstream complications, such as in-stent restenosis (ISR) or late stent thrombosis.[12–14] Because of the need for better visualization and improved understanding of the anatomic alterations that occur during PCI, intravascular ultrasound (IVUS) emerged as a valuable adjunct to conventional angiography.

ADVANTAGES OF INTRAVASCULAR ULTRASOUND

The use of IVUS as an adjunct imaging modality offers several advantages over conventional angiography. Compared with the 2-dimensional luminal silhouette created during angiography, IVUS offers visualization of the full circumference of the vessel wall. This improved visualization offers better characterization of coronary plaque via accurate assessment of the severity, length, morphology, and composition of the plaque. The direct cross-sectional view of the arterial wall produced by this technology provides higher sensitivity in detection of coronary artery disease. IVUS allows the operator to reliably detect complex coronary lesions, dissections, small thrombi, positive arterial wall remodeling during early atherosclerosis, and even diffuse advanced disease within the vessel wall that are otherwise challenging to detect only under angiographic guidance.[15]

In addition, IVUS offers more precise stent deployment during PCI by ensuring proper expansion, length, and apposition of the stent. Multiple studies have demonstrated the importance of these measures during PCI. Two major predictors of ISR and stent thrombosis include stent underexpansion and "geographic miss."[16,17] Smaller intrastent minimum lumen area (MLA) results from stent-underexpansion, whereas the concept of

"geographic miss" refers to residual plaque edge that remains uncovered after stent deployment. Multiple analyses have shown that adjunctive use of IVUS during PCI resulted in larger stent sizes, greater final angiographic minimum lumen diameter (MLD), and larger minimum stent area.[18,19] When compared with dilation under angiographic guidance, the use of IVUS resulted in additional stent postdilation in as high as 80% of the cases.[20] All of these findings may be attributed to more accurate assessment of stent geometry, as visualized under IVUS guidance. IVUS-guided PCI has also been shown to use less contrast during stent deployment, which is advantageous in patients with renal insufficiency and in prevention of contrast-induced nephropathy.[21,22] Finally, perhaps one of the major benefits of IVUS-guided stenting is that the enhanced information from IVUS imaging may convince the operator that the result is already optimal, and that more intervention is no longer necessary. As the saying goes, "The enemy of 'good' is 'better'"; problems of inappropriate intervention may be averted by using IVUS imaging.

TECHNIQUE AND BASIC MEASUREMENTS

The IVUS catheter diameter ranges from 2.6 to 3.5 French with a miniaturized ultrasound transducer at its end, which is advanced over a guidewire and positioned to analyze the target lesion. High ultrasound frequencies, usually between 20 and 60 MHz, are used to provide grayscale images from the backscatter amplitude of the signal as the transducer rotates at 1800 rpm. Instead of a mechanically rotating transducer, images can be obtained with a synthetic aperture, but the image quality is not equal to the mechanically rotating transducer devices. Standard catheter delivery technique is used for IVUS examination, whereby the target coronary artery is cannulated, the IVUS probe is slowly advanced over the guidewire, and motorized or manual pullback is performed to record the desired segment.[23]

A normal arterial appearance is generated as a result of an abrupt change in acoustic impedance at the tissue interface within the trilaminar vessel wall. The first interface observed is at the border between blood and the leading edge of intima that appears bright. The second interface occurs at the external elastic membrane (EEM), which comprises the junction between media and adventitia. The muscle layer of the tunica media has a sonolucent appearance, whereas the outer adventitia layer appears bright or white on a grayscale image (Fig. 1).

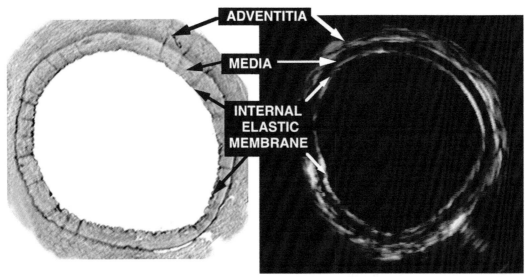

Fig. 1. IVUS image morphology of a nondiseased coronary artery (*right*) compared with its histologic cross-section (*left*). The 3 layers of the coronary artery are illustrated. The interface between the lumen and internal elastic membrane (inner layer) is the location of potential atherosclerosis. The dark sonolucent middle layer is the media, which outlines the size of the vessel in a nondiseased state. The outermost layer is the adventitia.

Planimetry is used to measure the atheroma area by subtracting the lumen area outlined by the intimal leading edge from the area surrounded by the EEM. The ratio between the plaque area measurement at the proximal reference area compared with the plaque area at the tightest lesion determines the significance of the stenosis. In general, 60% lumen area stenosis via IVUS measurements is considered significant.[24] Another measurement commonly performed is known as the MLA, which is an absolute value of the lumen area rather than a ratio compared with a reference segment. This measurement is made at the narrowest point in the epicardial vessel. Generally, MLA less than 4.0 mm² in the proximal epicardial vessels and less than 6.0 mm² in the left main vessel are considered significant.[25,26] A third measure of atheroma severity is the plaque burden. The plaque burden compares the total atheroma area at an individual cross-section divided by the total vessel area defined as the area subtended by the EEM. Studies have shown that total plaque burden and MLA are predictors of future clinical events.[27]

OPTIMIZATION OF STENT IMPLANTATION

The process of optimizing stent implantation begins during the preimplantation stage and continues during stent deployment as well as postimplantation. Before stent deployment, IVUS can be used to assess the lesion and surrounding anatomy, to create precise measurements of the reference segment, which further guides device selection and sizing of balloons and stents.[28] IVUS grayscale can also reveal important characteristics of the type of tissue that constitutes the atherosclerotic plaque (**Fig. 2**). IVUS is very sensitive to the presence of calcium and can reveal the relative hardness of a lesion, which may influence the choice of device, such as rotational atherectomy. During the stent deployment stage, IVUS guidance can assist with predilation, proper positioning of the balloon in relation to stent struts, and proper deployment of stents, thereby minimizing stent underexpansion or incomplete stent apposition. Last, after stent implantation, IVUS can aid in uncovering and treating complications, such as stent edge dissections, geographic mismatch, or plaque protrusion through the stent.

Several studies have evaluated the use of IVUS guidance on stent implantation, but definite guidelines regarding IVUS-guided stent optimization are lacking. Hence, stent optimization is often left to the discretion of the individual operator,[29] although generalized optimization criteria exist based on previous trials. For example, $(EEM^{ref}_{proximal} + EEM^{ref}_{distal})/2$ or EEM^{ref}_{distal} are 2 of the most common computations used to estimate the balloon diameter.[30,31] Similarly, IVUS criteria for optimal stent implantation, first established by the Multicenter Ultrasound Stenting In Coronaries Study investigators, includes MLA greater than 80% of the average reference lumen

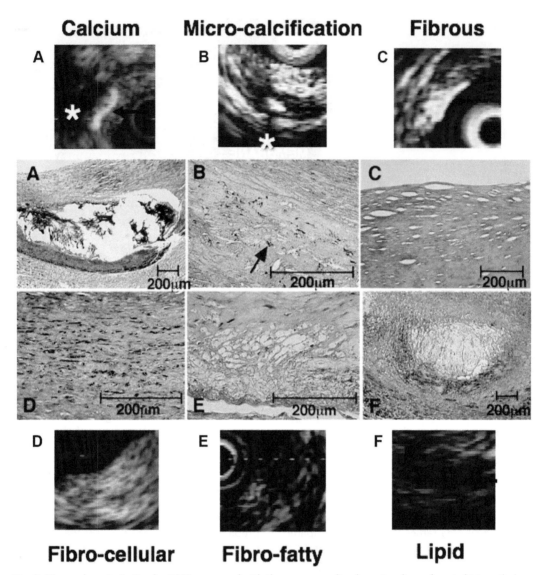

Fig. 2. Tissue characterization by IVUS compared with the corresponding hematoxylin and eosin histopathology. IVUS can be useful in detecting plaques of different morphologies, including plaque consisting of calcium (*A*), microcalcification (*B*), fibrous (*C*), fibrocellular (*D*), fibrofatty (*E*), and lipid-rich (*F*) material. Calcium deposits (*black arrows*) with IVUS appear as echogenic superficial reflections followed by an acoustic shadow (*asterisks*), both of which prevent thickness assessment.

area or greater than 90% of lumen area of the reference segment with the lowest lumen area.[32] By using the motorized transducer pullback method on IVUS, the distance between the distal and proximal landing zone can be measured, which estimates the optimal length for the stent to be deployed.[29] Complete stent apposition, minimal stent area (MSA) >90% of mean MLA[ref], or greater than 100% minimum MLA[ref] is usually considered one of many acceptable criteria for optimal stent expansion.[32] Evaluation of IVUS-guided stent expansion in the era of bare-metal stents (BMS) was evaluated by

Fitzgerald and colleagues[33] in the Can Routine Ultrasound Influence Stent Expansion study. The findings of this multicentered, randomized controlled trial showed that as compared with coronary angiography, addition of IVUS guidance was associated with larger MLD and MSA, which translated into clinically and statistically significant lower rates of target vessel revascularization (TVR). Gil and colleagues[34] showed similar findings in their multicenter, randomized, prospective trial, which demonstrated that, compared with angiographic guidance, IVUS-guided stent implantation resulted in the greatest lumen gain

(MLD) along with significant reduction in composite major adverse cardiac events (MACE). Robust evidence regarding superior stent expansion and apposition with IVUS optimization has been presented by other researchers as well.[35,36]

INTRAVASCULAR ULTRASOUND GUIDANCE DURING BARE-METAL AND DRUG-ELUTING STENT IMPLANTATION

During the era of BMS, the use of IVUS was first studied by Nakamura and colleagues. Although not powered for hard clinical endpoints, the investigators found that IVUS guidance resulted in larger minimum luminal diameter (MLD) during the index procedure and reduction in restenosis rates during the 6-month follow-up period.[20,37] In addition, by maximizing the lumen cross-sectional area, there was significantly less acute stent thrombosis such that the extended use of anticoagulation was no longer necessary. The lower incidence of acute stent thrombosis and freedom from extended use of anticoagulation revolutionized coronary artery stenting and lead to its general acceptance. Similar findings were suggested by a large meta-analysis of 8 randomized trials that demonstrated IVUS-guided BMS implantation was associated with lower rates of MACE.[38]

With the widespread use of drug-eluting stents (DES), which have a lower rate of restenosis compared with BMS,[39,40] there was concern that the use of IVUS guidance during PCI in the DES era would reap no additional benefit. These initial speculations were met with mixed results from several randomized controlled trials (Table 1). Jakabcin and colleagues[41] conducted a trial consisting of 210 patients who were randomized to DES implantation with or without IVUS guidance. At an 18-month follow-up, the investigators found that there was no significant difference in MACE or stent thrombosis between the 2 groups. A prospective, randomized trial of IVUS-guided compared with angiography-guided stent implantation in complex coronary lesions (AVIO) trial by Chieffo and colleagues[42] was a larger trial consisting of 284 patients with primary endpoint being improvement in postprocedure MLD. Secondary endpoints of this study were outcomes of MACE, TLR, TVR, myocardial infarction (MI), and stent thrombosis. The study demonstrated a benefit with IVUS guidance in regards to the primary outcome. However, no statistically significant difference was appreciated in the secondary outcomes, including MACE. The Impact of Intravascular Ultrasound Guidance on Outcomes of Xience Prime Stents in Long Lesions

(IVUS-XPL) was the largest, randomized, multicenter trial on this topic.[43] This trial enrolled 1400 patients with long coronary lesions, defined as ≥28 mm in length. At 1-year follow-up, IVUS guidance was superior to angiographic guidance in terms of TLR (2.5% vs 5.0%; hazard ratio [HR] = 0.51; confidence interval [CI] = 0.28–0.91; $P = .02$), whereas there was no significant difference in cardiac death and MI.

The Assessment of Dual Antiplatelet Therapy with Drug-Eluting Stents (ADAPT-DES) was a large study of ~8600 patients who received second-generation DES. ADAPT-DES was a prospective, multicenter, nonrandomized trial wherein the investigators performed a propensity-adjusted analysis to assess the relationship between IVUS use and clinical outcomes at 1-year follow-up. ADAPT-DES demonstrated superiority of IVUS-guided PCI compared with conventional angiography; the IVUS group demonstrated a significantly lower risk of stent thrombosis (0.6% vs 1.0%; HR = 0.40, CI = 0.21–0.73, $P = .003$), MI (2.5% vs 3.7%, HR = 0.66, CI = 0.49–0.88, $P = .004$), and composite MACE (3.1% vs 4.7%, HR = 0.70, CI = 0.55–0.88, $P = .002$) (Fig. 3).[44] The investigators noted that risk reduction was significant in all groups but was remarkably apparent in the patients with complex lesions or acute coronary syndrome presentation. The use of IVUS resulted in additional optimization during PCI as larger-sized stents/balloons, higher inflation pressures, and longer stents were used. Additional postdilation was also performed during PCI under IVUS guidance. Although favorable outcomes were applauded, critics noted the observational nature of the study along with the decision to use IVUS being left to the operator's discretion, thereby potentiating unmeasured confounders.

ADAPT-DES was followed by several well-conducted meta-analyses, which have brought further clarity to this subject by showing improvement in MLD and restenosis rates with IVUS-guided DES PCI[18,19,45,46] (Table 2). Elgendy and colleagues[47] conducted a meta-analysis of 7 randomized trials with 3200 patients treated with first- or second-generation DES. At a 15-month mean follow-up, patients in the IVUS-guided group experienced a significant reduction in risk of MACE (6.5% vs 10.3%; odds ratio = 0.60; CI = 0.46–0.77; $P<.0001$) because of reduction in TLR (4.1% vs 6.6%; $P<.0001$), whereas only a marginal reduction was seen in stent thrombosis (0.6% vs 1.3%; $P = .04$) and cardiovascular mortality (0.5% vs 1.2%; $P = .05$). In a patient level analysis of

Table 1
Randomized clinical trials comparing drug-eluting stent implantation with intravascular ultrasound guidance versus conventional angiographic guidance

Reference, Year	Design	Lesion Type	DES Type	1-y Outcome	MACE Definition	Follow-up (mo)	Results
Zhang et al,[46] 2015	Single center	Small lesion[a]	Second generation	Postprocedure in lesion MLD	Cardiac death, MI, or TVR	12	Significant reduction in MACE with IVUS
IVUS-XPL4,[43] 2015	Multicenter	Long coronary lesions	Second generation	MACE	Cardiac death, TLR-related MI, or TLR	12	MACE was lower in IVUS-guided group
CTO-IVUS,[53] 2015	Multicenter	CTOs	Second generation	Cardiac death	Cardiac death, MI, or TVR	12	No significant difference in cardiac death between the 2 groups
AIR-CTO,[54] 2015	Multicenter	CTOs	First/second generation[e]	In-stent LLL	Death, MI, TLR, or ST	12	In-stent LLL was significantly lower in the IVUS-guided group
Tan et al,[61] 2015	Single center	Unprotected left main coronary lesions	First generation	MACE	Cardiac death, MI, or TLR	24	IVUS-guided group had significantly lower rate of MACE
RESET,[80] 2013	Multicenter	Long coronary lesions[b]	Second generation	MACE	Cardiac death, MI, ST, or TVR	12	No statistically significant differences between rates of MACE between the 2 groups
AVIO,[42] 2013	Multicenter	Complex lesions[c]	First generation	Postprocedure in lesion MLD	Cardiac death, MI, or TVR	24	Statistically significant benefit in postprocedure MLD was seen with IVUS guidance
HOME DES IVUS,[41] 2010	Single center	Complex coronary lesion or complex patients' characteristics[d]	First generation	MACE	Death, MI, TLR	18	No significant difference between both groups in terms of MACE

Abbreviations: CTO, chronic total occlusion; LLL, late lumen loss; ST, stent thrombosis; TLR, target lesion revascularization.
[a] Small vessel (diameter 2.25–2.75 mm).
[b] Implanted stent greater than 28 mm in length.
[c] Bifurcations, long lesions, CTOs, or small vessels.
[d] Lesion type B2 and C according to the American Heart Association, proximal left anterior descending artery, left main disease, reference vessel diameter less than 2.5 mm, lesion length greater than 20 mm, ISR, insulin-dependent diabetes mellitus, and acute coronary syndrome.
[e] 76% first generation, and 24% second generation.

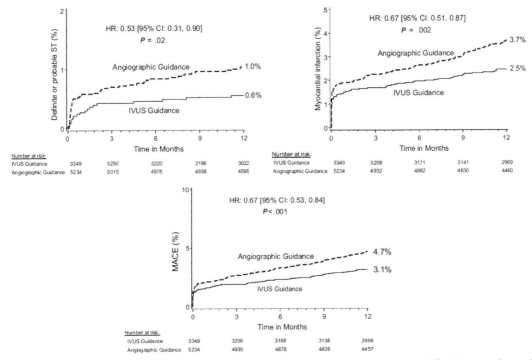

Fig. 3. IVUS versus angiographic guidance: time-to-event curves for stent thrombosis (*top left*), MI (*top right*), and MACE (*bottom*) within 1-year follow-up period. (*From* Witzenbichler B, Maehara A, Weisz G, et al. Relationship between intravascular ultrasound guidance and clinical outcomes after drug-eluting stents: the assessment of dual antiplatelet therapy with drug-eluting stents (ADAPT-DES) study. Circulation 2014;129:468; with permission.)

3 randomized controlled trials including 2345 patients who underwent second-generation DES implantation,[48] use of IVUS was associated with a reduction in risk of composite cardiac death, MI, and stent thrombosis when compared with conventional angiography (0.4% vs 1.2%, $P = .04$). The risk reduction in MI remained even at 1-year follow-up. A meta-regression analysis of 14 randomized trials showed that benefit of IVUS guidance was enhanced for longer lesions. For every 10-mm increase in lesion length, IVUS-guided PCI resulted in a 19% decrease in MACE.[49]

INTRAVASCULAR ULTRASOUND GUIDANCE DURING PERCUTANEOUS CORONARY INTERVENTION OF CHRONIC TOTAL OCCLUSION

Several studies have investigated the role of IVUS during CTO interventions. IVUS-guided imaging via a side branch may visualize the entry site of the occluded cap, which may facilitate the CTO recanalization process.[50–52] The influence of IVUS guidance on clinical endpoints was first tested by researchers of The Chronic Total Occlusion Intervention with Drug-eluting Stents (CTO-IVUS) trial.[53] CTO-IVUS was a

multicenter, prospective, randomized controlled trial that compared CTO patients who underwent angiography-guided intervention versus IVUS-guided intervention after successful guidewire crossing. The primary endpoint was cardiac death, and the secondary endpoint was MACE, consisting of cardiac death, MI, and TVR. During the 12-month follow-up period, there was a significant reduction in MACE in the IVUS-guidance group compared with the angiography-guidance cohort (2.6% vs 7.1%, $P = .035$). Another large randomized controlled trial, The Angiographic and Clinical Comparisons of Intravascular Ultrasound Versus Angiography-Guided-Drug-Eluting Stent Implantation for Patients with Chronic Total Occlusion Lesions (AIR-CTO), was recently published.[54] Researchers evaluated differences in LLL after CTO intervention via angiography-guided versus IVUS-guided approach. The results of this trial were in line with lower rates of LLL, ISR, and stent thrombosis with an IVUS-guided approach compared with patients who underwent CTO PCI under conventional angiography guidance. Unfortunately, because of the small number of patients enrolled, improvement in these parameters did not translate to hard clinical outcomes, such as a reduction in MACE. Interpretation of

Table 2
Meta-analyses comparing stent implantation with intravascular ultrasound guidance versus conventional angiographic guidance

References	Patients	Studies	Stent Type	MACE	All-Cause Mortality	MI	ST	TLR	TVR
Bavishi et al,[78] 2017	3276	8 RCTs	DES	0.64 (0.51–0.80) P = .001	0.51 (0.23–1.12) P = .09	0.90 (0.58–1.41) P = .70	0.57 (0.26–1.23) P = .15	0.62 (0.45–0.86) P = .004	0.60 (0.42–0.87) P = .007
Elgendy et al,[47] 2016	3192	7 RCTs	DES	0.59 (0.46–0.76) P<.001	0.46 (0.21–1.00) P = .05	0.58 (0.030–1.11) P = .06	0.49 (0.24–0.99) P = .04	0.60 (0.43–0.84) P = .003	0.61 (0.41–0.91) P = .02
Shin et al,[48] 2016	2345	3[a] RCTs	DES	0.36 (0.13–0.99) P = .04	0.38 (0.10–1.42) P = .134	NR P = .026	0.50 (0.13–2.01) P = .320	0.61 (0.40–0.93) P = .02	NR
Steinvil et al,[79] 2016	31,283	7 RCTs and 18 observational	DES	0.76 (0.70–0.82) P<.001	0.62 (0.54–0.72) P<.001	0.67 (0.56–0.80) P<.001	0.58 (0.47–0.73) P<.001	0.77 (0.67–0.89) P = .005	0.85 (0.76–0.95) P = .005
Parise et al,[38] 2011	2193	7 RCTs	BMS	0.69 (0.49–0.97) P = .03	1.48 (0.81–2.69) P = .18	0.67 (0.34–1.34) P = .51	NR	0.66 (0.48–0.91) P = .004	NR

Data presented as relative risk of events and 95% confidence intervals after IVUS-guided versus conventional angiographic guided.
P value <.05 is significant.
Abbreviations: NR, not reported; RCTs, randomized control trials; ST, stent thrombosis.
[a] Patient level analysis.

the CTO anatomy and how to use IVUS to optimize the intervention requires experience and dedicated training. Along with this, future larger trials are needed to better determine the clinical outcomes with IVUS-guided PCI of CTO lesions.[55]

INTRAVASCULAR ULTRASOUND DURING LEFT MAIN CORONARY ARTERY INTERVENTIONS

Visualization and assessment of the left main coronary artery (LMCA) often present a unique challenge for several reasons. The LMCA may be a short vessel, which does not provide the observer with a normal segment for comparison. The aortic cusp may obscure visualization of the LMCA ostium under conventional angiography, and delineation of the distal LMCA is often hindered by the downstream bifurcation or trifurcation.[56] Thus, the addition of IVUS to conventional angiography for LMCA assessment has been studied with interest. The Evaluation of XIENCE versus Coronary Artery Bypass Surgery for Effectiveness of Left Main Revascularization (EXCEL) and Coronary Artery Bypass Grafting versus Drug Eluting Stent Percutaneous Coronary Angioplasty in the Treatment of Unprotected Left Main Stenosis (NOBLE) were 2 randomized trials that compared PCI using DES to coronary artery bypass surgery (CABG) for LMCA revascularization.[57,58] Although EXCEL found PCI and CABG to be comparable, the results of NOBLE favored CABG. The difference in outcomes of these trials may partially be explained by more frequent use of IVUS in the EXCEL trial, suggesting that IVUS-guided LMCA intervention may be superior to conventional angiography alone.[59] This speculation is supported by 2 midsize propensity-matched analyses, which were conducted in Spain and Korea.[26,60] These studies showed better outcomes with IVUS-guided unprotected LMCA PCI compared with conventional angiography. Superiority of IVUS-guided unprotected LMCA intervention was further confirmed by a small randomized trial by Tan and colleagues.[61] This study showed that the incidence of TLR was lower in the IVUS-guided unprotected LMCA PCI group and that IVUS guidance was an independent factor in survival free of MACE at a 2-year follow-up.

ROLE OF INTRAVASCULAR ULTRASOUND IN BIORESORBABLE VASCULAR SCAFFOLDS

Concern over the safety and efficacy of the ABSORB Bioresorbable Vascular Scaffold (BVS)

system has lingered since its inception. During initial analysis, the vascular response to the implantation of BVS was studied in detail via serial IVUS examinations, which showed stable findings and low rates of MACE.[62] However, data on long-term outcomes have revealed increased risk of adverse events and have shown statistically significant higher rates of MI and scaffold thrombosis.[63] In light of these negative findings, a warning was issued by the US Food and Drug Administration about these first-generation devices. Researchers have inquired as to whether this association with adverse outcomes may be attributed to the design and material of first-generation BVS or whether factors such as improper sizing, lesion preparation, or procedure optimization are to blame for device failure. To evaluate this further, Stone and colleagues[64] conducted an analysis after accounting for baseline patient and lesion characteristics. At 3-year follow-up, vessel sizing and operator technique were strongly associated with BVS-related clinical outcomes, despite accounting for other variables. The investigators demonstrated that aggressive predilation was associated with freedom from scaffold thrombosis, whereas optimal postdilation was associated with freedom from target lesion failure. These data underscore the importance of an optimal implantation strategy for BVS. The effect of optimal implantation technique on outcomes with BVS was further evaluated by another group of researchers, who showed that the risk of scaffold thrombosis is significantly lowered with an aggressive implantation strategy that included a low threshold for IVUS use.[65] In this prospective, 2-center, observational study of 264 patients with 400 lesions treated with BVS, IVUS was used in 86% of interventions. At 2-year follow-up, definite or probable scaffold thrombosis occurred in only 3 patients. Hence, BVS intervention requires specific implantation techniques, which is facilitated by IVUS. To ensure proper tissue coverage with the scaffolds, IVUS guidance can aid aggressive predilation, proper apposition, and adequate postdilation during BVS implantation.

INTRAVASCULAR ULTRASOUND AND OTHER INTRACORONARY IMAGING TECHNIQUES

Another modality that has gained interest in augmenting PCI is fractional flow reserve (FFR). This technology relies on a physiologic rather than visual assessment of coronary stenosis. Studies have demonstrated improvement in clinical outcomes and a reduction in MACE with FFR-guided PCI as compared with conventional angiography.[66] How FFR compares with IVUS-guided PCI also has been investigated. Correlation between FFR findings and IVUS parameters was found to be vessel dependent and particularly limited to small vessels with ischemic lesions.[67] When evaluating LMCA disease, Jasti and colleagues[68] demonstrated a strong correlation between IVUS parameters (MLD, MLA, area stenosis, and cross-sectional narrowing) and FFR's physiologic calculation. Based on their analysis, the investigators concluded that MLA of 5.8 mm^2 and MLD of 2.8 mm had the strongest correlation with FFR parameters consistent with physiologically significant stenosis. Similarly, for non-LMCA lesions, moderate correlation was found between FFR of less than 0.8 and MLA noted on IVUS.[69] A perfect correlation between these 2 modalities is not feasible given the need for different cutoff values depending on location of the lesion and amount of myocardium served by that particular vessel.[70]

LIMITATIONS OF INTRAVASCULAR ULTRASOUND

Although IVUS can be very useful in tissue characterization and defining anatomy, it has shortcomings. Compared with newer imaging modalities, such as optical coherence tomography (OCT), IVUS remains inferior in the detection of intracoronary thrombus. Similar echotextures on IVUS may represent different tissue components. For example, a sonolucent structure may represent a lipid-rich atheroma, but an intracoronary thrombus may also carry a similar hypoechoic appearance. In addition, artifacts can have an undesirable effect on ultrasound images, creating significant distortions in image quality.[71] Last, IVUS solely provides a visual assessment of the coronary anatomy, compared with FFR, which provides a physiologic evaluation.

TRENDS AND COST-EFFECTIVENESS OF INTRAVASCULAR ULTRASOUND USE

The rate of IVUS use with PCIs is low in the United States and other countries. A one-year analysis of the National Cardiovascular Data Registry reported rates as low as 20%, which has remained unchanged over the years.[72,73] In a 7-year analysis of the national inpatient sample, Elgendy and colleagues found the rate of IVUS use to be <9% during inpatient PCIs.[74] On the other hand, IVUS is used in a large percentage of catheterization procedures in Japan. It is hypothesized that

the lack of widespread use of IVUS may be due to the cost of equipment, increased procedural time, and the perception of not needing IVUS to obtain good angiographic results.[75] Alberti and colleagues[76] modeled the economic impact of IVUS and found it to be a fairly robust and economic strategy. The investigators reported the highest cost-effectiveness of IVUS would be in patients with at higher risk of restenosis (eg, diabetes, renal insufficiency, or those presenting with an acute coronary syndrome). Although the economic benefits of IVUS decrease after the first year, the benefits persist during longer follow-up.[19] It is important to note that based on the economic analysis, the incremental cost added by IVUS remained well within the Italian population's willingness-to-pay threshold. Finally, the economic analysis of IVUS was also assessed by researchers from Denmark who reported improved clinical outcomes as well as better cost-effectiveness with the use of IVUS in their single-center, prospective randomized trial.[77]

SUMMARY

Over the last 2 decades, there has been accumulating evidence to support the routine use of IVUS for PCI interventions, even in the era of second-generation DES. This benefit has been consistently confirmed in observational and randomized trials. Moreover, there is evidence to suggest a greater improvement in clinical outcomes when IVUS is used to guide complex PCIs (LMCA intervention, complicated coronary anatomy, longer lesions, or CTOs). In addition, studies have demonstrated that an IVUS-guided PCI approach appears cost-effective. Although fairly robust data demonstrate improvement in clinical and angiographic outcomes with IVUS-guided interventions, most operators are reluctant to adopt the regular use of IVUS during PCI, because of the perceived increase in procedural time, lack of operator expertise, and lack of conviction of the need for IVUS use.

REFERENCES

1. Levine GN, Bates ER, Blankenship JC, et al. 2011 ACCF/AHA/SCAI guideline for percutaneous coronary intervention. A report of the American College of Cardiology Foundation/American Heart Association Task Force on Practice Guidelines and the Society for Cardiovascular Angiography and Interventions. J Am Coll Cardiol 2011;58:e44–122.
2. Elgendy IY, Kumbhani DJ, Mahmoud AN, et al. Routine invasive versus selective invasive strategies for non-ST-elevation acute coronary syndromes: an

updated meta-analysis of randomized trials. Catheter Cardiovasc Interv 2016;88:765–74.

3. White CW, Wright CB, Doty DB, et al. Does visual interpretation of the coronary arteriogram predict the physiologic importance of a coronary stenosis? N Engl J Med 1984;310:819–24.

4. Kern MJ, Donohue TJ, Aguirre FV, et al. Assessment of angiographically intermediate coronary artery stenoses using the Doppler flow wire. Am J Cardiol 1993;71:26D–33D.

5. Topol EJ, Nissen SE. Our preoccupation with coronary luminology. The dissociation between clinical and angiographic findings in ischemic heart disease. Circulation 1995;92:2333–42.

6. Zir LM. Observer variability in coronary angiography. Int J Cardiol 1983;3:171–3.

7. Galbraith JE, Murphy ML, Desoyza N. Coronary angiogram interpretation: interobserver variability. JAMA 1981;240:2053–9.

8. Isner JM, Kishel J, Kent KM. Accuracy of angiographic determination of left main coronary arterial narrowing. Circulation 1981;63:1056–61.

9. Nallamothu BK, Spertus JA, Lansky AJ, et al. Comparison of clinical interpretation with visual assessment and quantitative coronary angiography in patients undergoing percutaneous coronary intervention in contemporary practice: the Assessing Angiography (A2) project. Circulation 2013;127:1793–800.

10. Grodin CM, Dyrda I, Pasternac A, et al. Discrepancies between cineangiographic and postmortem findings in patients with coronary artery disease and recent myocardial revascularization. Circulation 1974;49:703–9.

11. Roberts WC, Jones AA. Quantitation of coronary arterial narrowing at necropsy in sudden coronary death. Am J Cardiol 1979;44:39–44.

12. Stone GW, Moses JW, Ellis SG, et al. Safety and efficacy of sirolimus and paclitaxel-eluting coronary stents. N Engl J Med 2007;356:998–1008.

13. Holmes DR, Kereiakes DJ, Laskey WK, et al. Thrombosis and drug-eluting stents: an objective appraisal. J Am Coll Cardiol 2007;50:109–18.

14. Fujii K, Mintz GS, Kobayashi Y, et al. Contribution of stent underexpansion to recurrence after sirolimus-eluting stent implantation for in-stent restenosis. Circulation 2004;109:1085–8.

15. Kastelein JJ, de Groot E. Ultrasound imaging techniques for the evaluation of cardiovascular therapies. Eur Heart J 2008;29:849–58.

16. Fujii K, Carlier SG, Mintz GS, et al. Stent underexpansion and residual reference segment stenosis are related to stent thrombosis after sirolimus-eluting stent implantation: an intravascular ultrasound study. J Am Coll Cardiol 2005;45:995–8.

17. Sonoda S, Morino Y, Ako J, et al, SIRIUS Investigators. Impact of final stent dimensions on long-term results following sirolimus-eluting stent implantation: serial intravascular ultrasound analysis from the sirius trial. J Am Coll Cardiol 2004;43:1959–63.

18. Jang JS, Song YJ, Kang W, et al. Intravascular ultrasound-guided implantation of drug-eluting stents to improve outcome: a meta-analysis. JACC Cardiovasc Interv 2014;7:233–43.

19. Ahn JM, Kang SJ, Yoon SH, et al. Meta-analysis of outcomes after intravascular ultrasound-guided versus angiography guided drug-eluting stent implantation in 26,503 patients enrolled in three randomized trials and 14 observational studies. Am J Cardiol 2014;113:1338–47.

20. Nakamura S, Colombo A, Gaglione A, et al. Intracoronary ultrasound observations during stent implantation. Circulation 1994;89:2026–34.

21. Ali ZA, Karimi Galougahi K, Nazif T, et al. Imaging- and physiology-guided percutaneous coronary intervention without contrast administration in advanced renal failure: a feasibility, safety, and outcome study. Eur Heart J 2016;37:3090–5.

22. Mariani J Jr, Guedes C, Soares P, et al. Intravascular ultrasound guidance to minimize the use of iodine contrast in percutaneous coronary intervention: the MOZART (minimizing contrast utilization with IVUS guidance in coronary angioplasty) randomized controlled trial. JACC Cardiovasc Interv 2014;7:1287–93.

23. Nissen SE, Yock P. Intravascular ultrasound novel pathophysiological insights and current clinical applications. Circulation 2001;103:604–16.

24. Mintz GS, Nissen SE, Anderson WD, et al. American College of Cardiology Clinical Expert Consensus Document on Standards for Acquisition, Measurement and Reporting of Intravascular Ultrasound Studies (IVUS): a report of the American College of Cardiology Task Force on Clinical Expert Consensus Documents. J Am Coll Cardiol 2001;37:1478–92.

25. Abizaid AS, Mintz GS, Mehran R, et al. Long-term follow-up after percutaneous transluminal coronary angioplasty was not performed based on intravascular ultrasound findings: importance of lumen dimensions. Circulation 1999;100:256–61.

26. de la Torre Hernandez JM, Baz Alonzo JA, Gomez Hospital JA, et al. Clinical impact of intravascular ultrasound guidance in drug-eluting stent implantation for unprotected left main coronary artery disease: pooled analysis at the patient-level of 4 registries. JACC Cardiovasc Interv 2014;7:244–54.

27. Stone GW, Maehara A, Lansky AJ, et al. A prospective natural-history study of coronary atherosclerosis. N Engl J Med 2011;364:226–35.

28. Mintz GS. IVUS in PCI guidance – Part II In American College of Cardiology Expert Analysis. 2016. Available at: http://www.acc.org/latest-in cardiology/articles/2016/06/13/10/01/ivus-in-pci-guidance/. Accessed November 12, 2017.

29. Yoon HJ, Hur SH. Optimization of stent deployment by intravascular ultrasound. Korean J Intern Med 2012;27:30–8.

30. Schiele F, Meneveau N, Gilard M, et al. Intravascular ultrasound-guided balloon angioplasty compared with stent. Immediate and 6-month results of the multicenter, randomized balloon equivalent to stent study (BEST). Circulation 2003;107:545–51.

31. Frey AW, Hodgson JM, Müller CH, et al. Ultrasound-guided strategy for provisional stenting with focal balloon combination catheter: results from the randomized strategy for intracoronary ultrasound-guided PTCA and stenting (SIPS) trial. Circulation 2000;102:2497–502.

32. de Jaegere P, Mudra H, Figulla H, et al. Intravascular ultrasound-guided optimized stent deployment. Immediate and 6 months clinical and angiographic results from the Multicenter Ultrasound Stenting In Coronaries Study (MUSIC Study). Eur Heart J 1998;19:1214–23.

33. Fitzgerald PJ, Oshima A, Hayase M, et al. Final results of the Can Routine Ultrasound Influence Stent Expansion (CRUISE) study. Circulation 2000;102:523–30.

34. Gil RJ, Pawlowski T, Dudek D, et al, Investigators of Direct Stenting vs Optimal Angioplasty Trial (DIPOL). Comparison of angiographically guided direct stenting technique with direct stenting and optimal balloon angioplasty guided with intravascular ultrasound. The multicenter, randomized trial results. Am Heart J 2007;154:669–75.

35. Russo RJ, Silva PD, Teirstein PS, et al. A randomized controlled trial of angiography versus intravascular ultrasound-directed bare-metal coronary stent placement (the AVID Trial). Circ Cardiovasc Interv 2009;2:113–23.

36. Oemrawsingh PV, Mintz GS, Schalij MJ, et al. Intravascular ultrasound guidance improves angiographic and clinical outcome of stent implantation for long coronary artery stenoses: final results of a randomized comparison with angiographic guidance (TULIP Study). Circulation 2003;107:62–7.

37. Albiero R, Rau T, Schluter M, et al. Comparison of immediate and intermediate-term results of intravascular ultrasound versus angiography-guided Palmaz-Schatz stent implantation in matched lesions. Circulation 1997;96:2997–3005.

38. Parise H, Maehara A, Stone GW, et al. Meta-analysis of randomized studies comparing intravascular ultrasound versus angiographic guidance of percutaneous coronary intervention in predrug-eluting stent era. Am J Cardiol 2011;107:374–82.

39. Bavry AA, Bhatt DL. Appropriate use of drug-eluting stents: balancing the reduction in restenosis with the concern of late thrombosis. Lancet 2008;371:2134–43.

40. Palmerini T, Benedetto U, Biondi-Zoccai G, et al. Long-term safety of drug-eluting and bare-metal stents: evidence from a comprehensive network meta-analysis. J Am Coll Cardiol 2015;65:2496–507.

41. Jakabcin J, Spacek R, Bystron M, et al. Long-term health outcome and mortality evaluation after invasive coronary treatment using drug eluting stents with or without the IVUS guidance. Randomized control trial. HOME DES IVUS. Catheter Cardiovasc Interv 2010;75:578–83.

42. Chieffo A, Latib A, Caussin C, et al. A prospective, randomized trial of intravascular-ultrasound guided compared to angiography guided stent implantation in complex coronary lesions: the AVIO trial. Am Heart J 2013;165:65–72.

43. Hong S, Kim B, Shin D, et al, for the IVUS-XPL Investigators. Effect of intravascular ultrasound–guided vs angiography-guided everolimus-eluting stent implantation the IVUS-XPL randomized clinical trial. JAMA 2015;314(20):2155–63.

44. Witzenbichler B, Maehara A, Weisz G, et al. Relationship between intravascular ultrasound guidance and clinical outcomes after drug-eluting stents: the assessment of dual antiplatelet therapy with drug-eluting stents (ADAPT-DES) study. Circulation 2014;129:463–70.

45. Zhang Y, Farooq V, Garcia-Garcia HM, et al. Comparison of intravascular ultrasound versus angiography-guided drug-eluting stent implantation: a meta-analysis of one randomised trial and ten observational studies involving 19,619 patients. EuroIntervention 2012;8:855–65.

46. Zhang YJ, Pang S, Chen XY, et al. Comparison of intravascular ultrasound guided versus angiography guided drug eluting stent implantation: a systematic review and meta-analysis. BMC Cardiovasc Disord 2015;15:153.

47. Elgendy IY, Mahmoud AN, Elgendy AY, et al. Outcomes with intravascular ultrasound-guided stent implantation: a meta-analysis of randomized trials in the era of drug-eluting stents. Circ Cardiovasc Interv 2016;9:e003700.

48. Shin DH, Hong SJ, Mintz GS, et al. Effects of intravascular ultrasound-guided versus angiography-guided new-generation drug-eluting stent implantation: meta-analysis with individual patient-level data from 2,345 randomized patients. JACC Cardiovasc Interv 2016;9:2232–9.

49. Elgendy IY, Mahmoud AN, Elgendy AY, et al. Does the baseline coronary lesion length impact outcomes with IVUS-guided percutaneous coronary intervention? J Am Coll Cardiol 2016;68:569–70.

50. Ito S, Suzuki T, Ito T, et al. Novel technique using intravascular ultrasound-guided guidewire cross in coronary intervention for uncrossable chronic total occlusions. Circ J 2004;68:1088–92.

51. Matsubara T, Murata A, Kanyama H, et al. IVUS-guided wiring technique: promising approach for the chronic total occlusion. Catheter Cardiovasc Interv 2004;61:381–6.

52. Ochiai M, Ogata N, Araki H, et al. Intravascular ultrasound guided wiring for chronic total occlusions. Indian Heart J 2006;58:15–20.

53. Kim BK, Shin DH, Hong MK, et al, CTO-IVUS Study Investigators. Clinical impact of intravascular ultrasound-guided chronic total occlusion intervention with zotarolimus-eluting versus biolimus-eluting stent implantation: randomized study. Circ Cardiovasc Interv 2015;8:e002592.

54. Tian NL, Gami SK, Ye F, et al. Angiographic and clinical comparisons of intravascular ultrasound-versus angiography-guided drug-eluting stent implantation for patients with chronic total occlusion lesions: two-year results from a randomised AIR-CTO study. EuroIntervention 2015;10:1409–17.

55. Galassi AR, Sumitsuji S, Boukhris M, et al. Utility of intravascular ultrasound in percutaneous revascularization of chronic total occlusions: an overview. JACC Cardiovasc Interv 2016;9:1979–91.

56. Mintz GS, Guagliumi G. Intravascular imaging in coronary artery disease. Lancet 2017;390:793–809.

57. Stone GW, Sabik JF, Serruys PW, et al, on behalf of the EXCEL Trial Investigators. Everolimus-eluting stents or bypass surgery for left main coronary artery disease. N Engl J Med 2016;375:2223–5.

58. Mäkikallio T, Holm NR, Lindsay M, et al, NOBLE study investigators. Percutaneous coronary angioplasty versus coronary artery bypass grafting in treatment of unprotected left main stenosis (NOBLE): a prospective, randomised, open-label, non-inferiority trial. Lancet 2016;388:2743–52.

59. Mahmoud AN, Elgendy IY, Mentias A, et al. Percutaneous coronary intervention or coronary artery bypass grafting for unprotected left main coronary artery disease. Catheter Cardiovasc Interv 2017;90:541–52.

60. Park SJ, Kim YH, Park DW, et al, MAIN-COMPARE Investigators. Impact of intravascular ultrasound guidance on long-term mortality in stenting for unprotected left main coronary artery stenosis. Circ Cardiovasc Interv 2009;2:167–77.

61. Tan Q, Wang Q, Liu D, et al. Intravascular ultrasound guided unprotected left main coronary artery stenting in the elderly. Saudi Med J 2015;36:549–53.

62. Serruys PW, Ormiston J, van Geuns RJ, et al. A polylactide bioresorbable scaffold eluting everolimus for treatment of coronary stenosis: 5-year follow-up. J Am Coll Cardiol 2016;67:766–76.

63. Mahmoud AN, Barakat AF, Elgendy AY, et al. Long-term efficacy and safety of Everolimus-eluting Bioresorbable vascular scaffolds versus Everolimus-eluting metallic stents: a meta-analysis of randomized trials. Circ Cardiovasc Interv 2017;10:e005286.

64. Stone GW, Abizaid A, Onuma Y, et al. Effect of technique on outcomes following bioresorbable vascular scaffold implantation: analysis from the ABSORB trials. J Am Coll Cardiol 2017;70(23):2863–74.

65. Tanaka A, Latib A, Kawamoto H, et al. Clinical outcomes of a real-world cohort following bioresorbable vascular scaffold implantation utilising an optimised implantation strategy. EuroIntervention 2017;12:1730–7.

66. Tonino PA, De Bruyne B, Pijls NH, et al. Fractional flow reserve versus angiography for guiding percutaneous coronary intervention. N Engl J Med 2009;360:213–24.

67. Costa MA, Sabate M, Staico R, et al. Anatomical and physiologic assessments in patients with small coronary artery disease: final results of the physiologic and anatomical evaluation prior to and after stent implantation in small coronary vessels (PHANTOM) trial. Am Heart J 2007;153:296.e1-7.

68. Jasti V, Ivan E, Yalamanchili V, et al. Correlations between fractional flow reserve and intravascular ultrasound in patients with an ambiguous left main coronary artery stenosis. Circulation 2004;110:2831–6.

69. Waksman R, Legutko J, Singh J, et al. FIRST: fractional flow reserve and intravascular ultrasound relationship study. J Am Coll Cardiol 2013;61:917–23.

70. Koo BK, Yang HM, Doh JH, et al. Optimal intravascular ultrasound criteria and their accuracy for defining the functional significance of intermediate coronary stenoses of different locations. JACC Cardiovasc Interv 2011;4:803–11.

71. ten Hoff H, Korbijn A, Smith TH, et al. Imaging artifacts in mechanically driven ultrasound catheters. Int J Card Imaging 1989;4:195–9.

72. Dattilo PB, Prasad A, Honeycutt E, et al. Contemporary patterns of fractional flow reserve and intravascular ultrasound use among patients undergoing percutaneous coronary intervention in the United States: insights from the National Cardiovascular Data Registry. J Am Coll Cardiol 2012;60:2337–9.

73. Mahtta D, Mahmoud AN, Mojadidi MK, et al. Intravascular ultrasound—guided percutaneous coronary intervention: an updated review. Cardiovasc Innov Appl 2017. https://doi.org/10.15212/CVIA.2017.0029.

74. Elgendy IY, Ha LD, Elbadawi A, et al. Temporal trends in inpatient use of intravascular imaging among patients undergoing percutaneous coronary intervention in the United States. JACC Cardiovasc Interv 2018.

75. Elgendy IY, Choi C, Bavry AA. The impact of fractional flow reserve on revascularization. Cardiol Ther 2015;4:191–6.

76. Alberti A, Giudice P, Gelera A, et al. Understanding the economic impact of intravascular ultrasound (IVUS). Eur J Health Econ 2016;17:185–93.

77. Gaster AL, Slothuus Skjoldborg U, Larsen J, et al. Continued improvement of clinical outcome and cost effectiveness following intravascular ultrasound guided PCI: insights from a prospective, randomised study. Heart 2003;89:1043–9.

78. Bavishi C, Sardar P, Chatterjee S, et al. Intravascular ultrasound-guided vs angiography-guided drug-eluting stent implantation in complex coronary lesions: meta-analysis of randomized trials. Am Heart J 2017;185:26–34.

79. Steinvil A, Zhang Y-J, Lee SY, et al. Intravascular ultrasound-guided drug-eluting stent implantation: an updated meta-analysis of randomized control trials and observational studies. Int J Cardiol 2016;216:133–9.

80. Kim JS, Kang TS, Mintz GS, et al. Randomized comparison of clinical outcomes between intravascular ultrasound and angiography-guided drug-eluting stent implantation for long coronary artery stenoses. JACC Cardiovasc Interv 2013;6:369–76.

Algorithmic Approach for Optical Coherence Tomography–Guided Stent Implantation During Percutaneous Coronary Intervention

Evan Shlofmitz, DO[a,b,c], Richard A. Shlofmitz, MD[b],
Keyvan Karimi Galougahi, MD, PhD[a], Hussein M. Rahim, MD[a],
Renu Virmani, MD[d], Jonathan M. Hill, MD[e,f], Mitsuaki Matsumura, BS[c],
Gary S. Mintz, MD[c], Akiko Maehara, MD[a,c], Ulf Landmesser, MD[g],
Gregg W. Stone, MD[a,c], Ziad A. Ali, MD, DPhil[a,b,c,*]

KEYWORDS

- Optical coherence tomography • Intravascular imaging • Percutaneous coronary intervention
- Stent

KEY POINTS

- Intravascular imaging plays a key role in optimizing outcomes for percutaneous coronary intervention (PCI).
- Optical coherence tomography (OCT) utilizes a user-friendly interface and provides high-resolution images.
- Incorporating a standardized, algorithmic approach when using OCT allows for precision PCI.
- OCT can be used as part of daily practice in all stages of an intervention: baseline lesion assessment, stent selection, and stent optimization.

INTRODUCTION

Angiography remains the primary method of imaging the coronary arteries to guide clinical decision making and treatment strategy in percutaneous coronary intervention (PCI). Angiography has several well recognized limitations, however. Angiography provides 2-D lumenography of a complex 3-D structure, neglecting the vessel wall in which atherosclerosis manifests. Adjunctive use of intravascular imaging may overcome some of these limitations and can provide clinical benefit. Multiple meta-analyses, including both registries and randomized trials,

---

Disclosure Statement: See last page of article.
[a] Center for Interventional Vascular Therapy, Division of Cardiology, NewYork-Presbyterian Hospital, Columbia University Medical Center, 161 Fort Washington Avenue, New York, NY 10032, USA; [b] Department of Cardiology, St. Francis Hospital, 100 Port Washington Boulevard, Suite 105, Roslyn, NY 11576, USA; [c] Clinical Trials Center, Cardiovascular Research Foundation, 1700 Broadway 9th Floor, New York, NY 10019, USA; [d] CVPath Institute, 19 Firstfield Road, Gaithersburg, MD 20878, USA; [e] London Bridge Hospital, 2nd Floor, St Olaf House, London SE1 2PR, UK; [f] Department of Cardiology, King's College Hospital, Denmark Hill, London, SE5 9RS, UK; [g] Department of Cardiology, Charité – Universitätsmedizin Berlin, Hindenburgdamm 30, Berlin 12200, Germany
* Corresponding author. Center for Interventional Vascular Therapy, Division of Cardiology, NewYork-Presbyterian Hospital, Columbia University Medical Center, New York, NY 10019.
E-mail address: zaa2112@columbia.edu

Intervent Cardiol Clin 7 (2018) 329–344
https://doi.org/10.1016/j.iccl.2018.03.001
2211-7458/18/© 2018 Elsevier Inc. All rights reserved.

have suggested the benefit of intravascular imaging-guided PCI in reducing death, target lesion failure, major adverse cardiac events (MACEs), and stent thrombosis.[1–5]

Optical coherence tomography (OCT) is an imaging modality initially developed for ophthalmologic use and later adopted for intracoronary imaging. OCT utilusesizes light-based technology to obtain 360° cross-sectional images of a coronary artery with a continuous pullback image of an arterial segment with resolution not previously available. Compared with intravascular ultrasound (IVUS), which incorporates soundwave technology and has a resolution of 40 μm to 200 μm, OCT has a higher axial resolution of 10 μm to 20 μm. The improved resolution allows accurate identification of the three layers of the normal arterial wall, delineation of plaque morphology, and highly sensitive identification of post-PCI complications.[1–8] Moreover, the improved resolution reduces interobserver and intraobserver variability of measurements on OCT compared with IVUS, facilitating operator training.[9]

Despite accumulating data supporting the benefit of intravascular imaging on PCI outcomes, adoption has been limited, especially for OCT. Central among the reasons for restricted adoption has been the lack of a standardized protocol for using intravascular imaging in contemporary practice. This review provides an overview on how to use OCT, summarizing the data supporting its clinical utility in the setting of a simple, user-friendly, "how to" OCT algorithm that may be implemented universally in the catheterization laboratory.

Optical Coherence Tomography Set-up

The only OCT catheter currently available in the United States for commercial use is the Dragonfly OPTIS imaging catheter (Abbott, St. Paul, Minnesota) (**Fig. 1**). Additional OCT imaging catheters are widely available outside the United States that differ in their utilization of optical frequency domain imaging but are largely based on the same fundamental technology. The Dragonfly OPTIS catheter is a rapid exchange, dual-lumen imaging catheter with a tip that tapers to a 2.7-F diameter. It is compatible with a 6-F or larger guiding catheter and offers fast acquisition, with automated pullback 2 sedonds to 3 seconds in duration. There are 3 radiopaque markers on the imaging catheter: The distal marker located 4 mm from the tip of the catheter, the lens marker located 2 mm proximal to the lens, and a third marker located 50 mm proximal to the lens marker (length marker) that can be used to approximate the imaging segment.

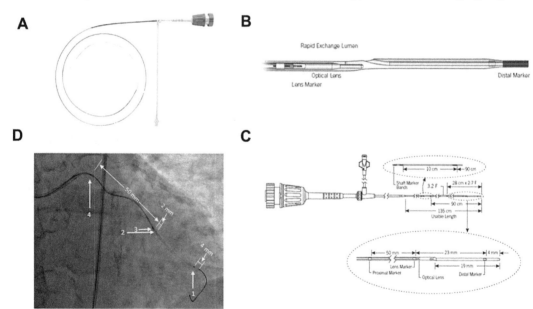

Fig. 1. Dragonfly OPTIS OCT imaging catheter. (*A*) The Dragonfly OPTIS catheter; (*B*) depiction of the longitudinal cross-section of the catheter; (*C*) dimensions of catheter components; and (*D*) angiogram with the Dragonfly imaging catheter with 3 radiopaque markers: (1) distal marker: a fixed marker located 4 mm from the tip of the catheter; (2) lens marker: located 2 mm proximal to the lens; (3) optical lens: located 2 mm distal to the lens marker; (4) proximal length marker: located 50 mm proximal to the lens and can be used to approximate the imaging segment. ([*A–C*] *From* Dragonfly, OPTIS and St. Jude Medical are trademarks of St. Jude Medical, LLC or its related companies. *Reproduced with permission of* St. Jude Medical, ©2018. All rights reserved.)

The length marker and lens markers are affixed to the imaging core and move proximally during the pullback, with the tip marker remaining stationary. The Dragonfly OPTIS imaging catheter connects to the OPTIS or the ILUMIEN OCT imaging system through the drive motor and optical controller. The newest generation of the technology, the OPTIS integrated system, allows for OCT-angiography coregistration (Fig. 2).

The pullback length can be selected as either 54 mm (high-resolution mode, 10 frames/mm) or 75 mm (survey mode, 5 frames/mm). The survey mode allows for a greater length of imaging of the artery while using less contrast with a shorter pullback time; thus, this should be preferentially selected as the default mode for initial lesion assessment. The OCT catheter should be advanced to the area of interest on standby mode under fluoroscopic guidance. "Live image" should be enabled several millimeters distal to the edge of the angiographic lesion. The guide catheter should be engaged in a fashion identical to preparation for PCI, ensuring that contrast delivery fully opacifies the coronary artery, which in turn ensures high-quality OCT image acquisition essential for image interpretation. "Deep-seating" of the guide is not advised, because the force of injection may lead to disengagement of the guide catheter resulting in poor-quality images. OCT-angiography coregistration may be optimized by selecting angiographic views, which avoid vessel overlap or foreshortening. Pullback can be triggered manually or automatically, with automatic set as the default. Automatic pullback is triggered when the lens detects a significant change in luminal pixilation in the peri-catheter zone. Flush medium is necessary to clear the lumen of blood to allow imaging acquisition by the OCT near-infrared light, which is conventionally achieved with radiocontrast medium. Prior to initial flush clearance, intracoronary nitroglycerin should be administered to minimize catheter related spasm. Flush clearance allows for clear differentiation between the lumen and vessel structure, allowing for automatic detection of the lumen

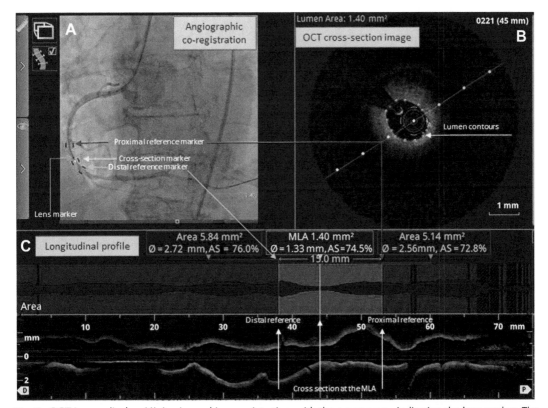

Fig. 2. OCT image display. (A) Angiographic coregistration, with the green arrow indicating the lens marker. The white bar represents the lens. The proximal reference is indicated by the red marker, distal reference by the blue marker and location of the OCT cross-section by the yellow marker. (B) OCT cross-section image obtained from location of the lens (*white bar* [A]), with lumen contours in green highlighting the lumen and automated measurement of the lumen area. (C) Longitudinal image of the vessel with markers at the designated proximal and distal references, with automated measurement of the MLA and proximal and distal reference area, mean diameter, and length.

contour and its dimensions, which are not possible by IVUS. To acquire an image, the "enable" button on the OCT drive motor and optical controller or console is pressed to calibrate and then pressed again; flush medium is then injected while cine-angiography is performed. The OPTIS OCT system then reconstitutes 3 sets of images: (1) cross-sectional; (2) "L-mode," which provides automated luminal measurements, including mean diameters and minimum luminal area (MLA); and (3) longitudinal (see Fig. 2).

Angiographic coregistration may be performed after image acquisition by selecting (1) an area of the vessel distally and (2) a point within the guide on the displayed angiographic image. The tracking-based coregistration is displayed as a white dot at the area of interest that closely coregisters to the cross-sectional OCT image (to within 1 mm). Manual measurement features include the ability to measure diameter, area, and length at the area of interest. In the settings menu, or by clicking the magnifying glass while hovering over the OCT cross-section, the field of view (zoom) may be adjusted within a range of 5 mm to 10 mm, permitting full visualization for larger vessels including the left main coronary artery. Bifurcation mode can be useful for assessing side branches at major bifurcation points as part of procedural planning.

CLINICAL EVIDENCE

There is currently a paucity of data supporting the routine use of OCT in PCI to improve clinical outcomes. The utility of OCT in clinical practice, however, has been established through several important studies (Table 1). In the Centro per la Lotta contro l'Infarto-Optimisation of Percutaneous Coronary Intervention (CLI-OPCI)[10] and CLI-OPCI II[11] studies, OCT was associated with improved outcomes compared with angiography alone. The OPUS-CLASS[12] study demonstrated the superior accuracy and reproducibility of dimension measurements using OCT compared with IVUS. The Observational Study of Optical Coherence Tomography in Patients Undergoing Fractional Flow Reserve and Percutaneous Coronary Intervention (ILUMIEN) I[7] study defined PCI optimization parameters with OCT and determined the impact of OCT guidance on decision making by physicians and on clinical events. This study demonstrated that pre-PCI OCT led to a change in treatment strategy in 57% of lesions and post-PCI OCT led to further stent optimization in 27% of lesions.

ILUMIEN II[13] was a retrospective, post hoc comparison of OCT-guided compared with IVUS-guided stent expansion, and demonstrated a similar degree of stent expansion with the 2 modalities. ILUMIEN III[8] was a landmark randomized controlled trial comparing OCT-guided, IVUS-guided, and angiography-guided PCI. The ILUMIEN III study demonstrated that stent diameter sizing decisions based on the use of the external elastic lamina (EEL) diameter measurement (rather than historical use of the lumen) was feasible and resulted in similar stent expansion compared with IVUS-guided stenting.[8] Prior to ILUMIEN III, OCT-guided diameter measurements and stent sizing had been based on lumen measurements, resulting in smaller final minimum stent areas (MSAs) achieved compared with EEL-based measurements on IVUS. Finally, in ILUMIEN III, OCT was substantially more sensitive than IVUS and angiography in detecting and preventing major dissections and areas of stent malapposition. For a more comprehensive overview of the current evidence, readers are referred to a recent review.[14]

GUIDELINES

Current guidelines reflect the limited long-term outcomes data available for OCT-guided PCI. American College of Cardiology/American Heart Association/Society for Cardiovascular Angiography and Interventions guidelines for PCI have not established the appropriate role for OCT in routine clinical decision making.[15,16] The European Society of Cardiology guidelines in myocardial revascularization recommend, however, that OCT should be considered in patients to understand the mechanism of stent failure (class IIa, level of evidence C), with OCT used in selected patients to optimize stent implantation (class IIb, level of evidence C).[17,18]

PERCUTANEOUS CORONARY INTERVENTION OPTIMIZATION

The use of treatment algorithms can lead to improved outcomes while helping to standardize clinical practice.[19] Following a protocol for incorporating OCT into clinical practice provides a practical approach to ensure optimization of each intervention. The authors describe an 8-step algorithm to achieve OCT-guided PCI optimization focusing on preintervention lesion assessment, stent deployment, and post-stent assessment and optimization (Fig. 3). Importantly, OCT should be performed at baseline (pre-PCI) and after stent implantation. If

Trial	N	Study Design	Outcome
Table 1			
Key optical coherence tomography trials			
Habrara et al,[32] 2012	70 patients	Randomized, single center; superiority of IVUS vs OCT	OCT-guidance based on lumen dimensions resulted in smaller final stent expansion compared with IVUS guidance.
CLI-OPCI,[10] 2012	670 patients	Observational comparison of OCT-guided PCI vs matched angio-guided PCI	OCT guidance was associated with a significantly lower rate of events at 1 y.
OPUS-CLASS,[12] 2013	100 patients	Prospective, multicenter comparison of OCT, IVUS, and phantom models	OCT provides accurate and reproducible quantitative measurements of coronary dimensions.
CLI-OPCI II,[11] 2015	832 patients, 1002 lesions	Retrospective, multicenter analysis of end-procedural OCT	Suboptimal stent deployment based on OCT criteria was associated with increased MACE.
ILUMIEN I,[7] 2015	418 patients, 467 stenoses	Prospective, nonrandomized, observational study	Physician decision making was affected by OCT imaging prior to PCI in 57% and post-PCI in 27% of all cases. OCT-guided PCI resulted in smaller lumen areas than angiography-guided PCI.
ILUMIEN II,[13] 2015	940 patients	Post hoc matched-paired analysis of ILUMIEN and ADAPT-DES patients	OCT and IVUS guidance resulted in similar stent expansion.
ILUMIEN III,[8] 2016	450 patients	Randomized, controlled multicenter trial comparing OCT-guided, IVUS-guided, and angiography-guided PCI	A specific EEL-based stent optimization strategy was feasible in the majority of cases and resulted in a MSA similar to that in IVUS-guided PCI.
DOCTORS,[63] 2016	240 patients	Randomized, multicenter comparison of OCT-guided PCI vs angiography-guided PCI	Higher postprocedure FFR in OCT-guided arm, with similar procedural complications. OCT led to PCI optimization in 50% of OCT-guided cases.
OPINION,[64] 2017	829 patients	Randomized, noninferiority of OCT vs IVUS	Target vessel failure by OCT guidance using lumen-based stent sizing was noninferior to IVUS guidance using vessel diameter for stent sizing.

Abbreviation: FFR, fractional flow reserve.

optimal stent expansion criteria are not met (described later), measures should be taken to further optimize the stent, followed by repeat OCT to verify an acceptable result.

PREPROCEDURAL ASSESSMENT

OCT performed prior to PCI is useful to characterize plaque morphology and extent, to guide lesion preparation strategies, and to determine the optimal stent diameter and length. Although

OCT image acquisition is most commonly acquired using contrast medium flush, overall use of contrast medium with OCT guidance can be comparable or even less than angiography-guided PCI. Because OCT provides a tomographic view of the coronary artery, diagnostic angiography in multiple projections may be minimized. For diagnostic angiography, 3 views may be sufficient to determine the presence or absence of a target lesion—left anterior oblique-cranial for the right coronary artery

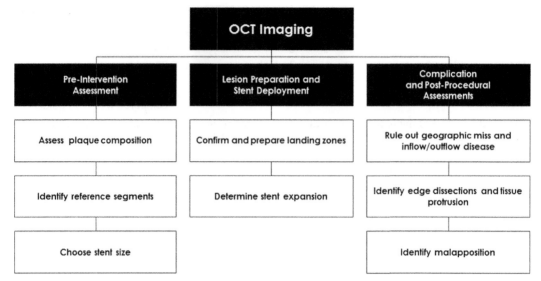

Fig. 3. Algorithm for precision PCI.

and anterior/posterior-caudal and anterior/posterior-cranial for the left coronary artery. If no target lesion has been identified, further tailored angiography may be performed; however, if a target vessel is identified, further diagnostic angiography should be performed during target vessel OCT-image acquisition (preferably using angiographic coregistration), allowing 3-D tomographic assessment of the coronary artery.

OCT allows delineation of the layers of the normal artery wall (Fig. 4). A simple algorithmic approach to reading OCT images that allows for accurate and reproducible image interpretation can be implemented based on recognition of these layers and the principles of near-infrared light. Visualization of the EEL and adventitia in the entire vessel circumference of a cross-section represents either a normal artery segment or a fibrous plaque. On the contrary, light attenuation in any region of the plaque implies pathology—most commonly either lipid or calcium. If light attenuation is recognized, the next step is to determine the location of the light attenuation, that is, whether it is originating from the lumen or within the vessel wall. The magnitude of attenuation then allows for the determination of the plaque characteristics (Fig. 5).

Plaque composition guides lesion preparation strategy. For largely fibrous and lipidic lesions without calcification, predilatation may

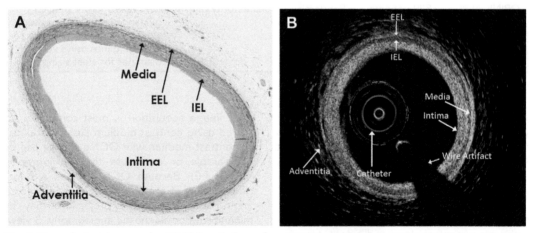

Fig. 4. Normal artery topography. (A) Histopathology of a normal coronary artery segment with clear delineation of intima, media, and adventitia. (B) OCT image of a normal coronary artery segment with key structures labeled. IEL, internal elastic lamina.

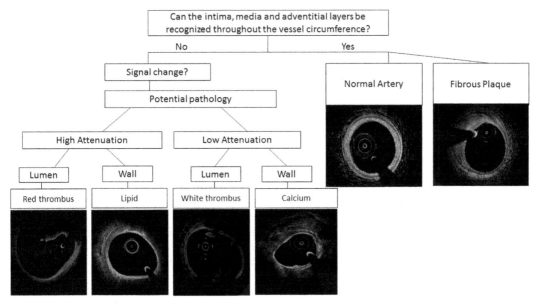

Fig. 5. Identification of plaque composition.

be unnecessary, and direct stenting may be considered. On the contrary, vessel preparation for calcific plaque, known to be underdiagnosed by angiography,[20] may be tailored by OCT guidance. Diagnosis of not only the presence, but extent, of calcification is critical, because moderate/severe calcification is strongly predictive of target lesion revascularization and is an independent predictor of stent thrombosis.[21] The maximum arc of target lesion calcification is an important determinant of stent expansion and thus the MSA that can be achieved,[22] which is perhaps the single most important predictor of outcomes after drug-eluting stent implantation.[23–25] OCT is the imaging modality of choice to detect the presence and severity of calcification, because, unlike angiography or IVUS, OCT is able to not only differentiate deep from superficial calcium but also measure the thickness of calcium, a critical predictor of stent underexpansion.[26] Such comprehensive assessment of calcific plaque prior to PCI can guide strategy for vessel preparation and determine the treatment's effectiveness.[27,28] Calcium fracture after lesion preparation, which can be determined by OCT, has been shown to predict stent expansion in several recent studies.[29–31] As a general rule, the authors recommend atherectomy rather than balloon predilatation for lesion preparation in the presence of severe calcification.

As described previously, the light-attenuating properties of lipid and calcium may prohibit the identification of the EEL.

Habara and colleagues[32] reported greater than 270° visibility of the EEL in only 62.9% of reference segments identified as normal by angiography; however, in ILUMIEN III greater than 180° of the reference segment EEL (the threshold required to determine stent diameter) could be visualized by OCT in 85% of cases by the sites and 95% of cases by the OCT core laboratory within 5 mm of the original angiographically selected reference segment. Greater than 180° EEL could be visualized by IVUS in 83% of cases by the sites and 100% of cases by the IVUS core laboratory, suggesting the utility of OCT and IVUS in this regard are similar, despite the prevailing dogma. Although OCT is the only intravascular imaging modality truly able to detect a thin-cap fibroatheroma,[33] the precursor lesion to most cases of plaque thrombosis, the clinical utility of this capability is currently uncertain. Nonetheless, avoiding reference segments with large lipid burdens, in particular those with thin-cap fibroatheroma, is advisable given the association of edge problems with both stent thrombosis and MACE.[23,34–42] If lipid in the reference segment cannot be avoided, the authors recommend covering the entire lipidic region with a stent, rather than ending the stent in the middle of a lipid-rich plaque.

OCT is the most accurate imaging modality to measure vessel dimensions, which is useful to select balloon and stent diameters. Historically, most operators used OCT luminal dimensions to guide stent sizing,[10–12] leading to a disadvantage compared with EEL-based or midwall-based guidance by IVUS. Furthermore, when using identical sizing strategies in the same vessel (luminal, midwall, or EEL diameters) with OCT and IVUS, OCT yields smaller MSAs compared with IVUS because IVUS dimensions overestimate the true size by approximately 10% (unlike OCT, which is highly precise).[13] As a result, OCT is disadvantaged in achieving comparable stent sizes to IVUS in 2 ways: first assizing is commonly based on luminal measurements, compared with the vessel wall by IVUS, and second as consequence of IVUS overestimating dimensions. Because OCT has been shown more accurate and precise than IVUS for dimensional measurements, the authors recently investigated the utility of EEL-guided stent sizing by OCT. In the ILUMIEN III: OPTIMIZE PCI study, which randomized 450 patients to OCT-guided, IVUS-guided, or angiography-guided PCI,[14] an EEL-based stent sizing strategy resulted in similar MSA to that of IVUS-guided PCI with a trend toward larger MSA compared with angiography guidance and fewer untreated post-PCI complications. Achieving the maximal stent diameter safely is an essential goal of PCI, as small differences in stent diameter lead to large increases in stent area with proportionate benefit on PCI outcomes.[43] An EEL-based

algorithm for OCT-guided stent sizing is shown in **Fig. 6**, and an example of OCT-guided stent sizing is shown in **Fig. 7**.

STENT DEPLOYMENT

Precise stent deployment at the intended segments can be aided by OCT-angiography coregistration to improve the accuracy of stent placement and minimize geographic miss (goal <1 mm).[44,45] After stent deployment, stent expansion can be easily assessed using automated measures (**Fig. 8**). By placing markers that limit the area of interest bounding the proximal and distal edges of the stent, the MSA and percent stent expansion are automatically measured and highlighted (**Fig. 9**). Several criteria for optimal stent expansion have been previously described.[46] The Multicenter Ultrasound Stenting in Coronaries study criteria, based on IVUS, sought an in-stent MLA greater than or equal to 80% of the average reference lumen area with symmetric stent expansion.[47] The IVUS-XPL criteria required the MSA to be greater than or equal to the distal reference lumen area.[48] In ILUMIEN III, to account for natural vessel tapering, the stented segment was divided in half, with a goal of reaching an MSA in the proximal and distal stent of at least 90%

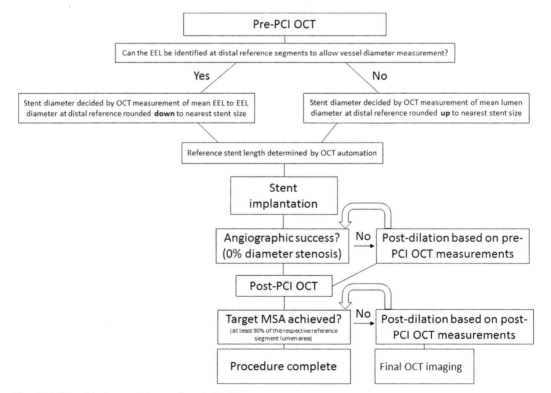

Fig. 6. OCT-guided stent sizing and optimization.

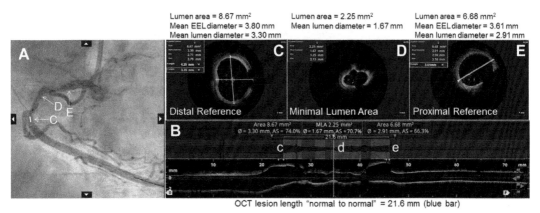

Lumen area = 8.67 mm²   Lumen area = 2.25 mm²   Lumen area = 6.68 mm²
Mean EEL diameter = 3.80 mm   Mean lumen diameter = 1.67 mm   Mean EEL diameter = 3.61 mm
Mean lumen diameter = 3.30 mm   Mean lumen diameter = 2.91 mm

OCT lesion length "normal to normal" = 21.6 mm (blue bar)

Fig. 7. Pre-PCI OCT with proximal and distal reference images. (1) Identify angiographic reference segments (A). (2) OCT lumen profile (B), identify segments with the largest lumen area within the reference segments (C – distal, E -proximal). (3) If the EEL can be identified, such that a vessel diameter measurement can be made, the reference segment cross-section is appropriate. If not, the reference segment area (±5 mm from the initially selected cross-section) should be perused to find a cross-section that allows EEL measurement. Only if the EEL cannot be used to measure vessel diameter should the lumen diameter be used for stent sizing. In this case, at the distal reference segment (C, coregistered with the angiogram C in [A] and lumen profile c in [B]) automated measures (green text) displays reference lumen area and min, max, and mean lumen diameter. Approximately 360° degrees of EEL is visualized, allowing multiple measurements of EEL for stent sizing. The measured EEL diameters of the distal reference segment were (white line) 4.25 mm and (blue line) 3.35 mm, resulting in a mean EEL diameter of 3.8 mm. The MLA (D, coregistered with the angiogram D in panel A and lumen profile d in panel B) by automated measures (green) was 2.25 mm². At the proximal reference segment (E, co-registered with the angiogram E [A and lumen profile e [B]) automated measures (green text) displays reference lumen area and min, max, and mean lumen diameter. Approximately 180° of EEL is visualized, allowing a single measurement of EEL for stent sizing. The measured EEL diameter of the proximal reference segment (white) was 3.61 mm. Note a mean EEL diameter could not be calculated because only 1 EEL measurement could be made. The smallest EEL diameter from both distal and proximal reference segments was 3.61 mm (distal reference) and per protocol this was rounded down to the nearest 0.25 mm; thus, a 3.5 mm diameter stent was chosen. (4) The stent length is determined. In this case, the distance from distal reference cross-section C (coregistered with the angiogram C [A] and lumen profile c [B]) to the proximal reference (E, co-registered with the angiogram E [A] and lumen profile e [B]) was 21.6 mm, thus a 3.5-mm × 22-mm or 23-mm stent would be appropriate. (5) Plaque morphology is assessed. Play and peruse the OCT pullback, focusing on plaque morphology within the diseased segment, to guide lesion preparation strategy, if any. In this case there was no significant calcification, and no lesion preparation was planned before stenting.

of the respective reference segment lumen area.[8] As the only studied OCT-specific criteria, the authors currently recommend following this ILUMIEN III guideline.

With regard to stent deployment, for practical purposes, OCT is best used to overcome the limitations of angiography. Thus, if following stent implantation, there is angiographic evidence of stent underexpansion, attempts to correct the underexpansion should be performed prior to repeat OCT imaging (see Fig. 6). Nonetheless, if pre-PCI OCT was performed, these measurements should guide the postdilation strategy. In each half of the stent, postdilation should be performed with a noncompliant balloon sized to the respective reference EEL-EEL diameter (but not larger) at high pressures. If the EEL could not be visualized at the reference on the pre-PCI OCT, a noncompliant balloon upsized from the mean lumen diameter at high pressures should be used (upsize 0.25 mm if the mean

lumen diameter is <3 mm or upsize 0.5 mm if the mean lumen diameter is ≥3 mm). If the stent underexpansion is in the middle of a long stent (≥28 mm), an intermediate balloon size between the distal and proximal reference diameters may be used. Only then should postoptimization OCT be performed, and if stent underexpansion persists, the post-PCI OCT measurements should be used to guide further postdilation identical to that described previously. It is not uncommon for the vessel diameter to grow considerably after initial stent implantation, particularly at the distal reference, due to flow-mediated dilatation.

Achieving these goals for stent expansion may not be possible in all cases, and clinical judgment must be used to balance the benefit of optimal stent expansion with the risk of perforation. In general, the authors recommend that, when sizing to the EEL, postdilation balloons should not exceed the diameter of the EEL in

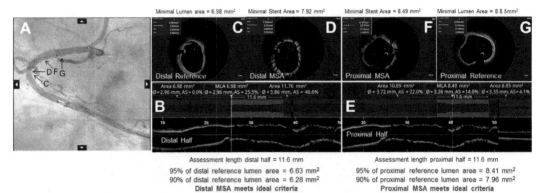

Fig. 8. Post-PCI OCT with assessment of stent expansion. (6) Angiographic assessment of the implanted stent is performed. In this case a 3.5 × 23 mm drug-eluting stent was implanted at 12 atm. Based on the angiographic appearance (A) of the distal stent (D), the stent was post-dilated along its mid and distal segments with a non-compliant balloon. The balloon diameter was selected based on the pre-PCI optical coherence tomography (OCT) measurements, which showed a mean external elastic lamina (EEL) diameter of 3.8 mm (see Fig. 7). Rounding down to the nearest balloon size, a 3.75 × 15 mm noncompliant balloon was inflated at 20 atm for 30 seconds to treat the under-expanded segment. (7) Angiographic assessment is repeated. In this case, angiography (not shown) revealed 0% residual diameter stenosis. (8) OCT is repeated to determine whether the previously under-expanded segment is now fully expanded. The stent length is divided in half, and criteria for MSA are assessed in each half. In this case, automated measures (B) identified the MLA of 6.98 mm^2 (yellow box) at the site of the unstented distal reference vessel. At the distal reference vessel (C), a small distal edge dissection was noted that was not treated. The MSA at the distal stent (D) was 7.92 mm^2, and thus optimal stent expansion was achieved ([1– (7.92/6.98)] ×100] = –13.5% area stenosis). (E) In the proximal half of the stented segment, automated measures measured an MSA (yellow box) of 8.49 mm^2 and a proximal reference lumen area of 8.85 mm^2, equating to a residual area stenosis (AS) of 4.1% ([1– (8.49/8.85)] ×100]), confirming criteria for MSA were met. (F) There was no significant tissue protrusion or malapposition at the site of proximal MSA. (G) At the proximal reference, there was minimal disease and no evidence of dissection.

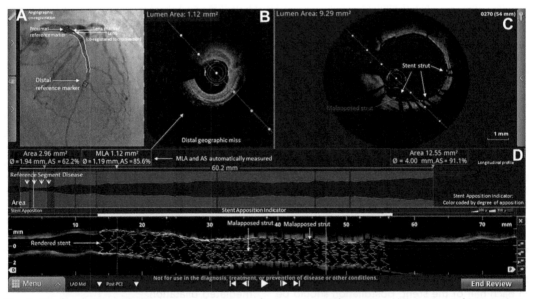

Fig. 9. Rendered stent with distal geographic miss and minor stent malapposition. (A) Angiographic coregistration, with the proximal reference marker, lens, lens marker, and distal reference marker labelled. Representative outlining of the location of the stent has been added to the angiographic image. (B) OCT cross-section image demonstrating distal geographic miss and automated measurement of the lumen area (1.12 mm^2). (C) OCT cross-section image demonstrating a malapposed stent strut (red arrow). (D) Longitudinal image of the vessel with rendered stent and markers at the designated proximal and distal references, with automated measurement of the MLA and proximal and distal reference area, mean diameter, area stenosis (AS), and length. The stent apposition indicator displays a bar the length of the stent, color coded by degree of apposition.

the respective halves of the stent, although iterative higher pressures inflated for longer durations may be instituted in an attempt to achieve stent expansion targets.

Assessment of Complications

Acute findings after stenting, including edge dissection, intramural hematoma, tissue protrusion, and incomplete stent apposition, are detectable on OCT with a higher sensitivity than compared with IVUS (Fig. 10).[8,49]

Geographic Miss and Inflow/Outflow Disease

Geographic miss can be easily confirmed with the automated lumen measurement profile and rendered stent features of OCT (see Fig. 9). After post-PCI OCT, the rendered stent selection should be activated. Visual inspection of the proximal and distal outflow (5 mm from the stent edges) allows for rapid determination of reference segment disease. If untreated reference segment disease is detected, the reference markers should be used to bound the respective reference segment and determine the MLA. If the MLA is less than or equal to 4.5 mm², an additional stent should be placed to correct the inflow or outflow unless there are anatomic reasons that the disease should not be covered (eg, diffuse distal disease or significant vessel tapering). Both inflow and outflow MLA less than 4.5 mm² have been shown to be strong predictors of poor PCI outcome.[11]

Edge Dissection

Stent edge complications are commonly observed with OCT that may not be identified by angiography alone.[8] An edge dissection is defined as a linear rim of tissue adjacent to a sent edge with a width greater than or equal to 200 μm.[10] Because stent edge dissection may lead to high rates of thrombosis and target lesion revascularization, OCT may be used to determine the severity of dissection to determine whether it requires correction.[41] Dissection depth (confined to the intima or deep within the media), location (proximal or distal), angle of dissection flap, length of the dissection, and the residual lumen area at the dissection site are key determinants.[8,10,50] Although contained intimal tears not reaching the media are likely benign, dissections that reach the media provide a tract for the development of intramural hematoma. In ILUMIEN III edge dissections were considered major by OCT when they extended greater than 60° in arc and greater than 3 mm in length based on data from the Assessment of Dual Antiplatelet Therapy With Drug Eluting Stents (ADAPT-DES) registry, which highlighted these measurements as predictors for stent thrombosis.[41] Previous studies have also shown that longer dissections may be less likely to heal spontaneously.[51] Any dissection with angiographic evidence of flow limitation or associated with an inadequate MLA (<4.5 mm²) should also be considered for correction.[11]

Tissue Protrusion

Tissue protrusion due either to thrombus or nonthrombotic plaque can be of varying importance based on its characteristics and morphology. Typically, tissue protrusion can be left untreated; however, in the situation of major tissue protrusion (effective MLA <5.5 mm² or reduction in flow area >10%) present, further postdilation, aspiration (in the case of thrombus), or additional short DES placement should be considered.[52] In particular, irregular protrusion, defined as protrusion of material with an irregular surface into the lumen between stent struts, has been identified as an independent predictor of 1-year device-oriented clinical end points and thus should be considered for treatment.[52] Tissue protrusion may have a greater detrimental effect in cases of acute coronary syndrome.[53]

Malapposition

A malapposition indicator is available on the OPTIS OCT system, highlighting areas of the stent that are separated from the vessel wall by greater than or equal to 0.2 mm (see

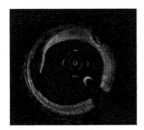
Edge dissection

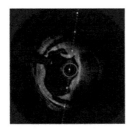
Major edge dissection

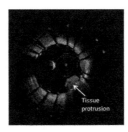
Tissue protrusion

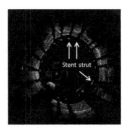
Stent malapposition

Fig. 10. Post-PCI complications.

Fig. 9). Although easily identified with OCT, the clinical consequences of acute strut malapposition remain controversial. Although multiple studies have demonstrated that acute malapposition is unrelated to adverse clinical outcomes,[54,55] a high frequency of malapposition is observed in cases of stent thrombosis.[56,57] In context, gross malapposition (>0.5 mm) (especially when continuous for >1 mm in length), malapposition in the setting of underexpansion (which may exacerbate turbulent flow), and proximal malapposition (which may hamper vessel re-entry) should be considered for correction.

Stent Failure

Use of OCT is particularly important in cases of stent failure (thrombosis or restenosis) to determine the etiology and determine the best treatment strategy. This is reflected in current European guidelines (class IIa, level of evidence C).[18] OCT demonstrates whether stent thrombosis is due to mechanical (eg, underexpansion) or other causes (eg, unrecognized edge dissection or major inflow/outflow obstruction). If the cause is not mechanical, optimal antiplatelet therapy may be readdressed using platelet reactivity assays. Similarly, with in-stent restenosis (ISR), OCT can provide insight into the mechanism of ISR, guiding the best treatment approach. OCT morphologic characteristics of ISR with second-generation DES differ for early and late presentation. Early ISR is associated with underexpansion, whereas neoatherosclerosis contributes more commonly to late ISR.[58] Stent underexpansion when diagnosed by OCT can be treated with high pressure balloon inflation, cutting or scoring balloons, laser, or atherectomy.[59–61] Multiple layers of well-expanded stents, where the predominant mechanism of ISR is recurrent neointimal hyperplasia, may be considered for brachytherapy.

CONTROVERSIES

Resistance to routine usage of OCT is largely based on the beliefs that OCT acquisition is cumbersome and time consuming, adds to the cost and contrast load, and provides an overload of information that is, hard to readily interpret in the catheterization laboratory. Like any new technology, there is a learning curve; however, with repeated use and incorporation of a standard algorithm, use of OCT can be a critical and often indispensable part of routine practice and improve patient outcomes. Although the OCT catheter has some cost, the additional

cost is often mitigated by several factors. OCT accurately determines the required length of a stent and its placement, possibly reducing the number of stents needed. Assessment of plaque composition may mitigate the need for predilation, and optimal stent sizing with OCT demonstration of adequate stent expansion may mitigate the need for postdilation. Contrast should always be used judiciously in the setting of renal insufficiency. Although dextran is used as an alternative flush agent for performing OCT, dextran is not recommended in patients with chronic kidney disease.[62]

FUTURE DIRECTIONS

Clinical evidence has demonstrated that OCT can improve procedural success and short-term outcomes. The upcoming, pivotal ILUMIEN IV study will evaluate long-term outcomes in patients with OCT-guided PCI in a global, multicenter, prospective, randomized controlled clinical trial.

SUMMARY

Accumulating evidence has demonstrated the improved clinical outcomes of imaging-guided PCI with IVUS. OCT offers improved resolution compared with IVUS with a more user-friendly interface, automated measurement capability, and seamless coregistration with angiography. An algorithmic approach to optimizing PCI with OCT ensures ease of use while potentially enhancing procedural success. Although the authors describe an 8-step algorithm that can be incorporated into daily practice, the exact protocol is less important than having a formalized and structured approach to OCT image acquisition and analysis, which may lead to higher rates of successful adoption by different operators. As with any new technology, there is an inherent learning curve, but with training and routine use, OCT can readily be performed in a time-effective manner and provide a wealth of complementary information to optimize PCI outcomes.

DISCLOSURE STATEMENT

E. Shlofmitz has served as a consultant for Cardiovascular Systems Inc. R.A. Shlofmitz has served as a speaker for Cardiovascular Systems Inc. R. Virmani receives research support from Abbott Vascular, BioSensors International, Biotronik, Boston Scientific, Medtronic, MicroPort Medical, OrbusNeich Medical, SINO Medical Technology, and Terumo Corporation; is a speaker for Merck; receives honoraria from

Abbott Vascular, Boston Scientific, Lutonix, Medtronic, and Terumo Corporation; and is a consultant for 480 Biomedical, Abbott Vascular, Medtronic, and W.L. Gore. J.M. Hill has served as a speaker and received honoraria and research grant support from Abbott Vascular. G.S. Mintz has served as a consultant for and received honoraria from Boston Scientific and ACIST Medical Systems; and received fellowship/grant support from Volcano, Boston Scientific, and InfraReDx. A. Maehara has received research grant support from Boston Scientific and Abbott Vascular; served as a consultant for Boston Scientific and OCT Medical Imaging; and received speaker fees Abbott Vascular. U. Landmesser has served as a consultant for and received honoraria from Abbott Vascular. G.W. Stone owns equity in SpectraWave. Z.A. Ali has received institutional research grant support from Abbott Vascular and Cardiovascular Systems Inc; and served as a consultant for Abbott Vascular, St. Jude Medical, Cardiovascular Systems Inc, and ACIST Medical Systems. All other authors have reported that they have no relationships relevant to the contents of this article to disclose.

REFERENCES

1. Zhang YJ, Pang S, Chen XY, et al. Comparison of intravascular ultrasound guided versus angiography guided drug eluting stent implantation: a systematic review and meta-analysis. BMC Cardiovasc Disord 2015;15(1):153.

2. Jang JS, Song YJ, Kang W, et al. Intravascular ultrasound-guided implantation of drug-eluting stents to improve outcome: a meta-analysis. JACC Cardiovasc Interv 2014;7(3):233–43.

3. Witzenbichler B, Maehara A, Weisz G, et al. Relationship between intravascular ultrasound guidance and clinical outcomes after drug-eluting stents: the assessment of dual antiplatelet therapy with drug-eluting stents (ADAPT-DES) study. Circulation 2014;129(4):463–70.

4. Elgendy IY, Mahmoud AN, Elgendy AY, et al. Outcomes with intravascular ultrasound-guided stent implantation: a meta-analysis of randomized trials in the era of drug-eluting stents. Circ Cardiovasc Interv 2016;9(4):e003700.

5. Ahn JM, Kang SJ, Yoon SH, et al. Meta-analysis of outcomes after intravascular ultrasound-guided versus angiography-guided drug-eluting stent implantation in 26,503 patients enrolled in three randomized trials and 14 observational studies. Am J Cardiol 2014;113(8):1338–47.

6. Tearney GJ, Regar E, Akasaka T, et al. Consensus standards for acquisition, measurement, and reporting of intravascular optical coherence tomography studies: a report from the International Working Group for Intravascular Optical Coherence Tomography Standardization and Validation. J Am Coll Cardiol 2012;59(12):1058–72.

7. Wijns W, Shite J, Jones MR, et al. Optical coherence tomography imaging during percutaneous coronary intervention impacts physician decision-making: ILUMIEN I study. Eur Heart J 2015;36(47):3346–55.

8. Ali ZA, Maehara A, Genereux P, et al. Optical coherence tomography compared with intravascular ultrasound and with angiography to guide coronary stent implantation (ILUMIEN III: OPTIMIZE PCI): a randomised controlled trial. Lancet 2016;388(10060):2618–28.

9. Fedele S, Biondi-Zoccai G, Kwiatkowski P, et al. Reproducibility of coronary optical coherence tomography for lumen and length measurements in humans (The CLI-VAR [Centro per la Lotta contro l'Infarto-VARiability] study). Am J Cardiol 2012;110(8):1106–12.

10. Prati F, Di Vito L, Biondi-Zoccai G, et al. Angiography alone versus angiography plus optical coherence tomography to guide decision-making during percutaneous coronary intervention: the Centro per la Lotta contro l'Infarto-Optimisation of Percutaneous Coronary Intervention (CLI-OPCI) study. EuroIntervention 2012;8(7):823–9.

11. Prati F, Romagnoli E, Burzotta F, et al. Clinical impact of OCT findings during PCI: The CLI-OPCI II study. JACC Cardiovasc Imaging 2015;8(11):1297–305.

12. Kubo T, Akasaka T, Shite J, et al. OCT compared with IVUS in a coronary lesion assessment: the OPUS-CLASS study. JACC Cardiovasc Imaging 2013;6(10):1095–104.

13. Maehara A, Ben-Yehuda O, Ali Z, et al. Comparison of stent expansion guided by optical coherence tomography versus intravascular ultrasound: the ILUMIEN II study (Observational Study of Optical Coherence Tomography [OCT] in patients undergoing Fractional Flow Reserve [FFR] and percutaneous coronary intervention). JACC Cardiovasc Interv 2015;8(13):1704–14.

14. Ali ZA, Karimi Galougahi K, Maehara A, et al. Intracoronary optical coherence tomography 2018: current status and future directions. JACC Cardiovasc Interv 2017;10(24):2473–87.

15. Levine GN, Bates ER, Bittl JA, et al. 2016 ACC/AHA guideline focused update on duration of dual antiplatelet therapy in patients with coronary artery disease: a report of the American College of Cardiology/American Heart Association Task Force on Clinical Practice Guidelines: an update of the 2011 ACCF/AHA/SCAI guideline for percutaneous coronary intervention, 2011 ACCF/AHA guideline

for coronary artery bypass graft surgery, 2012 ACC/AHA/ACP/AATS/PCNA/SCAI/STS guideline for the diagnosis and management of patients with stable ischemic heart disease, 2013 ACCF/AHA guideline for the management of ST-Elevation myocardial infarction, 2014 AHA/ACC guideline for the management of patients with Non-ST-Elevation acute coronary syndromes, and 2014 ACC/AHA guideline on perioperative cardiovascular evaluation and management of patients undergoing noncardiac surgery. Circulation 2016;134(10):e123–155.

16. Levine GN, Bates ER, Blankenship JC, et al. 2011 ACCF/AHA/SCAI guideline for percutaneous coronary intervention: a report of the American College of Cardiology Foundation/American Heart Association Task Force on Practice Guidelines and the Society for Cardiovascular Angiography and Interventions. Circulation 2011;124(23):e574–651.

17. Kolh P, Windecker S, Alfonso F, et al. 2014 ESC/EACTS guidelines on myocardial revascularization: the Task Force on Myocardial Revascularization of the European Society of Cardiology (ESC) and the European Association for Cardio-Thoracic Surgery (EACTS). Developed with the special contribution of the European Association of Percutaneous Cardiovascular Interventions (EAPCI). Eur J Cardiothorac Surg 2014;46(4):517–92.

18. Authors/Task Force Members, Windecker S, Kolh P, Alfonso F, et al. The task force on myocardila revascularization of the European Society of Cardiology (ESC) and the European Association for Cardio-Thoracic Surgery (EACTS). 2014 ESC/EACTS guidelines on myocardial revascularization. Eur Heart J 2014;35(37):2541–619.

19. Morris AH. Treatment algorithms and protocolized care. Curr Opin Crit Care 2003;9(3):236–40.

20. Mintz GS, Popma JJ, Pichard AD, et al. Patterns of calcification in coronary artery disease. A statistical analysis of intravascular ultrasound and coronary angiography in 1155 lesions. Circulation 1995;91(7):1959–65.

21. Genereux P, Madhavan MV, Mintz GS, et al. Ischemic outcomes after coronary intervention of calcified vessels in acute coronary syndromes. Pooled analysis from the HORIZONS-AMI (Harmonizing Outcomes With Revascularization and Stents in Acute Myocardial Infarction) and ACUITY (Acute Catheterization and Urgent Intervention Triage Strategy) trials. J Am Coll Cardiol 2014;63(18):1845–54.

22. Kobayashi Y, Okura H, Kume T, et al. Impact of target lesion coronary calcification on stent expansion. Circ J 2014;78(9):2209–14.

23. Fujii K, Carlier SG, Mintz GS, et al. Stent underexpansion and residual reference segment stenosis are related to stent thrombosis after sirolimus-eluting stent implantation: an intravascular ultrasound study. J Am Coll Cardiol 2005;45(7):995–8.

24. Sonoda S, Morino Y, Ako J, et al. Impact of final stent dimensions on long-term results following sirolimus-eluting stent implantation: serial intravascular ultrasound analysis from the sirius trial. J Am Coll Cardiol 2004;43(11):1959–63.

25. Fujii K, Mintz GS, Kobayashi Y, et al. Contribution of stent underexpansion to recurrence after sirolimus-eluting stent implantation for in-stent restenosis. Circulation 2004;109(9):1085–8.

26. Fujino A, Mintz G, Matsumura M, et al. TCT-28 a new optical coherence tomography-based calcium scoring system to predict stent underexpansion. J Am Coll Cardiol 2017;70(18):B12–3.

27. Karimi Galougahi K, Maehara A, Mintz GS, et al. Update on intracoronary optical coherence tomography: a review of current concepts. Curr Cardiovasc Imaging Rep 2016;9(6):16.

28. Barbato E, Shlofmitz E, Milkas A, et al. State of the art: evolving concepts in the treatment of heavily calcified and undilatable coronary stenoses - from debulking to plaque modification, a 40-year-long journey. EuroIntervention 2017;13(6):696–705.

29. Kubo T, Shimamura K, Ino Y, et al. Superficial calcium fracture after PCI as assessed by OCT. JACC Cardiovasc Imaging 2015;8(10):1228–9.

30. Maejima N, Hibi K, Saka K, et al. Relationship between thickness of calcium on optical coherence tomography and crack formation after balloon dilatation in calcified plaque requiring rotational atherectomy. Circ J 2016;80(6):1413–9.

31. Ali ZA, Brinton TJ, Hill JM, et al. Optical coherence tomography characterization of coronary lithoplasty for treatment of calcified lesions: first description. JACC Cardiovasc Imaging 2017;10(8):897–906.

32. Habara M, Nasu K, Terashima M, et al. Impact of frequency-domain optical coherence tomography guidance for optimal coronary stent implantation in comparison with intravascular ultrasound guidance. Circ Cardiovasc Interv 2012;5(2):193–201.

33. Kubo T, Tanaka A, Kitabata H, et al. Application of optical coherence tomography in percutaneous coronary intervention. Circ J 2012;76(9):2076–83.

34. Okabe T, Mintz GS, Buch AN, et al. Intravascular ultrasound parameters associated with stent thrombosis after drug-eluting stent deployment. Am J Cardiol 2007;100(4):615–20.

35. Liu X, Doi H, Maehara A, et al. A volumetric intravascular ultrasound comparison of early drug-eluting stent thrombosis versus restenosis. JACC Cardiovasc Interv 2009;2(5):428–34.

36. Choi SY, Witzenbichler B, Maehara A, et al. Intravascular ultrasound findings of early stent thrombosis after primary percutaneous intervention in acute myocardial infarction: a Harmonizing

Outcomes with Revascularization and Stents in Acute Myocardial Infarction (HORIZONS-AMI) substudy. Circ Cardiovasc Interv 2011;4(3):239–47.

37. Sakurai R, Ako J, Morino Y, et al. Predictors of edge stenosis following sirolimus-eluting stent deployment (a quantitative intravascular ultrasound analysis from the SIRIUS trial). Am J Cardiol 2005; 96(9):1251–3.

38. Liu J, Maehara A, Mintz GS, et al. An integrated TAXUS IV, V, and VI intravascular ultrasound analysis of the predictors of edge restenosis after bare metal or paclitaxel-eluting stents. Am J Cardiol 2009;103(4):501–6.

39. Costa MA, Angiolillo DJ, Tannenbaum M, et al. Impact of stent deployment procedural factors on long-term effectiveness and safety of sirolimus-eluting stents (final results of the multicenter prospective STLLR trial). Am J Cardiol 2008;101(12): 1704–11.

40. Kang SJ, Cho YR, Park GM, et al. Intravascular ultrasound predictors for edge restenosis after newer generation drug-eluting stent implantation. Am J Cardiol 2013;111(10):1408–14.

41. Kobayashi N, Mintz GS, Witzenbichler B, et al. Prevalence, features, and prognostic importance of edge dissection after drug-eluting stent implantation: an ADAPT-DES intravascular ultrasound substudy. Circ Cardiovasc Interv 2016;9(7):e003553.

42. Calvert PA, Brown AJ, Hoole SP, et al. Geographical miss is associated with vulnerable plaque and increased major adverse cardiovascular events in patients with myocardial infarction. Catheter Cardiovasc Interv 2016;88(3):340–7.

43. de Feyter PJ, Kay P, Disco C, et al. Reference chart derived from post-stent-implantation intravascular ultrasound predictors of 6-month expected restenosis on quantitative coronary angiography. Circulation 1999;100(17):1777–83.

44. Leistner DM, Riedel M, Steinbeck L, et al. Real-time optical coherence tomography coregistration with angiography in percutaneous coronary intervention-impact on physician decision-making: The OPTICO-integration study. Catheter Cardiovasc Interv 2017. [Epub ahead of print].

45. Koyama K, Fujino A, Yamamoto MH, et al. A prospective, single-Center, randomized study to assess whether co-registration of OCT and angiography can reduce geographic miss. Paper presented at: TCT 2016. Washington, DC, October 31, 2016.

46. Raber L, Ueki Y. Optical coherence tomography- vs. intravascular ultrasound-guided percutaneous coronary intervention. J Thorac Dis 2017;9(6):1403–8.

47. de Jaegere P, Mudra H, Figulla H, et al. Intravascular ultrasound-guided optimized stent deployment. Immediate and 6 months clinical and angiographic results from the Multicenter Ultrasound Stenting in Coronaries Study (MUSIC Study). Eur Heart J 1998; 19(8):1214–23.

48. Hong SJ, Kim BK, Shin DH, et al. Effect of intravascular ultrasound-guided vs angiography-guided everolimus-eluting stent implantation: The IVUS-XPL randomized clinical trial. JAMA 2015;314(20): 2155–63.

49. Kume T, Okura H, Miyamoto Y, et al. Natural history of stent edge dissection, tissue protrusion and incomplete stent apposition detectable only on optical coherence tomography after stent implantation - preliminary observation. Circ J 2012;76(3): 698–703.

50. Maehara A, Matsumura M, Mintz GS. Assessment and quantitation of stent results by intracoronary optical coherence tomography. Interv Cardiol Clin 2015;4(3):285–94.

51. Radu MD, Raber L, Heo J, et al. Natural history of optical coherence tomography-detected non-flow-limiting edge dissections following drug-eluting stent implantation. EuroIntervention 2014; 9(9):1085–94.

52. Soeda T, Uemura S, Park SJ, et al. Incidence and clinical significance of poststent optical coherence tomography findings: one-year follow-up study from a multicenter registry. Circulation 2015; 132(11):1020–9.

53. Prati F, Romagnoli E, Gatto L, et al. Clinical impact of suboptimal stenting and residual intrastent plaque/thrombus protrusion in patients with acute coronary syndrome: the CLI-OPCI ACS substudy (Centro per la Lotta Contro L'Infarto-Optimization of Percutaneous Coronary Intervention in Acute Coronary Syndrome). Circ Cardiovasc Interv 2016; 9(12):e003726.

54. Guo N, Maehara A, Mintz GS, et al. Incidence, mechanisms, predictors, and clinical impact of acute and late stent malapposition after primary intervention in patients with acute myocardial infarction: an intravascular ultrasound substudy of the Harmonizing Outcomes with Revascularization and Stents in Acute Myocardial Infarction (HORIZONS-AMI) trial. Circulation 2010;122(11):1077–84.

55. Steinberg DH, Mintz GS, Mandinov L, et al. Long-term impact of routinely detected early and late incomplete stent apposition: an integrated intravascular ultrasound analysis of the TAXUS IV, V, and VI and TAXUS ATLAS workhorse, long lesion, and direct stent studies. JACC Cardiovasc Interv 2010;3(5):486–94.

56. Souteyrand G, Amabile N, Mangin L, et al. Mechanisms of stent thrombosis analysed by optical coherence tomography: insights from the national PESTO French registry. Eur Heart J 2016;37(15): 1208–16.

57. Adriaenssens T, Joner M, Godschalk TC, et al. Optical coherence tomography findings in patients

with coronary stent thrombosis: a report of the PRESTIGE consortium (Prevention of Late Stent Thrombosis by an Interdisciplinary Global European Effort). Circulation 2017;136(11):1007–21.

58. Song L, Mintz GS, Yin D, et al. Characteristics of early versus late in-stent restenosis in second-generation drug-eluting stents: an optical coherence tomography study. EuroIntervention 2017;13(3):294–302.

59. Bastante T, Rivero F, Cuesta J, et al. Calcified neo-atherosclerosis causing "undilatable" in-stent restenosis: insights of optical coherence tomography and role of rotational atherectomy. JACC Cardiovasc Interv 2015;8(15):2039–40.

60. Alfonso F, Sandoval J, Nolte C. Calcified in-stent restenosis: a rare cause of dilation failure requiring rotational atherectomy. Circ Cardiovasc Interv 2012;5(1):e1–2.

61. Otsuka Y, Kasahara Y, Kawamura A. Use of SafeCut Balloon for treatment of in-stent restenosis of a previously underexpanded sirolimus-eluting stent with a heavily calcified plaque. J Invasive Cardiol 2007;19(12):E359–62.

62. Mailloux L, Swartz CD, Capizzi R, et al. Acute renal failure after administration of low-molecular weight dextran. N Engl J Med 1967;277(21):1113–8.

63. Meneveau N, Souteyrand G, Motreff P, et al. Optical coherence tomography to optimize results of percutaneous coronary intervention in patients with Non-ST-Elevation acute coronary syndrome: results of the multicenter, randomized DOCTORS study (Does Optical Coherence Tomography Optimize Results of Stenting). Circulation 2016;134(13):906–17.

64. Kubo T, Shinke T, Okamura T, et al. Optical frequency domain imaging vs. intravascular ultrasound in percutaneous coronary intervention (OPINION trial): one-year angiographic and clinical results. Eur Heart J 2017;38(42):3139–47.

Computed Tomography Fractional Flow Reserve to Guide Coronary Angiography and Intervention

Roshin C. Mathew, MS, MD[a], Matthew Gottbrecht, MD[a],
Michael Salerno, MD, PhD[a,b,c,d],*

KEYWORDS

• Fractional flow reserve (FFR) • Coronary computed tomography angiography (CTA) • CT-FFR
• Coronary artery disease

KEY POINTS

• Computed tomography (CT) fractional flow reserve (CT-FFR) uses coronary computed tomography angiography (CTA) images and computational fluid dynamics (CFD) to noninvasively simulate invasive FFR assessment.
• CT-FFR has higher specificity and positive predictive value as compared with visual analysis of coronary CTA stenosis using invasive FFR as the gold standard.
• In patients with a planned invasive coronary angiography, a strategy using CT-FFR as a gate-keeper to angiography is associated with a cost savings.
• In patients with a planned noninvasive assessment, CT-FFR is cost neutral and is associated with improvement in angina scores.
• Because of the high computational demand of CFD, machine-learning approaches are being developed as an alternative approach with the potential rapid evaluation of CT-FFR.

INTRODUCTION

More than a decade ago, the Fractional Flow Reserve versus Angiography for Guiding Percutaneous Intervention (FAME) trial led to a paradigm shift toward using the functional significance of a coronary lesion, as assessed by fractional flow reserve (FFR), rather than the anatomic severity of a coronary stenosis, to drive decision making regarding coronary revascularization. This multicenter trial, which randomized 1005 patients to angiographically guided percutaneous intervention (PCI) versus FFR-guided PCI (threshold FFR <0.8), demonstrated a 72% relative risk reduction of the composite endpoint of death, myocardial infarction, and repeat vascularization at 1 year of follow-up.[1] In FAME, only 35% of stenoses in the 50%

Disclosures: Dr M. Salerno receives research support from Siemens Healthineers and Astra Zeneca. Dr M. Salerno is a consultant to Locus Health and IBM Watson. Dr M. Salerno discloses the following research funding: NIH R01 HL131919. Commuted tomography angiography has played a significant role in coronary evaluation in the last decade.
[a] Department of Medicine, University of Virginia Health System, University of Virginia, 131 Hospital Drive, Suite 1031, Charlottesville, VA 22904, USA; [b] Department of Radiology and Medical Imaging, The Cardiovascular Imaging Center, University of Virginia Health System, 1215 Lee Street, Charlottesville, VA 22908, USA; [c] Department of Biomedical Engineering, University of Virginia Health System, 415 Lane Road, Room 2010, Charlottesville, VA 22908, USA; [d] Cardiovascular Division, University of Virginia Health System, 1215 Lee Street, PO Box 800158, Charlottesville, VA 22908, USA
* Corresponding author. Cardiovascular Division, University of Virginia Health System, 1215 Lee Street, PO Box 800158, Charlottesville, VA 22908.
E-mail address: ms5pc@virginia.edu

Intervent Cardiol Clin 7 (2018) 345–354
https://doi.org/10.1016/j.iccl.2018.03.008
2211-7458/18/© 2018 Elsevier Inc. All rights reserved.

to 70% range were functionally significant by FFR, demonstrating the discordance between hemodynamic significance and visual assessment of lesion severity.[2] The results after 2 and 5 years of follow-up confirmed long-term efficacy of an FFR-guided strategy.[3,4] The FAME 2 trial, which sought to assess the efficacy of medical therapy and stenting FFR-positive lesions versus opposed to medical therapy alone, was stopped prematurely because of a significant difference (4.3% in PCI group vs 12.2% in medical-therapy group, $P<.001$) in the primary endpoints between the 2 groups.[5] FFR currently has a class I recommendation in the 2014 Stable Ischemic Heart Disease guidelines and a score of "appropriate" in the 2017 appropriate use criteria for either PCI or coronary artery bypass grafting in patients with symptomatic physiologically significant stenosis (FFR <0.80).[6,7]

The necessity of improved methods for noninvasive evaluation of coronary artery disease (CAD) was highlighted in a retrospective study of the National Cardiovascular Data Registry, which demonstrated that only 37.6% of the 398,987 patients without known CAD who underwent coronary angiography had obstructive CAD, and having a positive noninvasive test only increased the rate of obstructive disease from 35% to 41%.[8] Over the past 2 decades, coronary computed tomography angiography (CTA) has emerged as a noninvasive methodology for evaluating the coronary arteries with a very high negative predictive value (NPV), and a moderate positive predictive value (PPV) as compared with invasive coronary angiography (ICA) and FFR.[9,10] Furthermore, CTA provides vessel-specific anatomic information, as opposed to other noninvasive modalities used to detect obstructive CAD.[11] Despite the strengths of CTA, the degree of stenosis identified using this modality does not necessarily correlate with the functional significance of the lesion as defined by invasive FFR. In some studies, lesions that were considered severe on CTA have been found to be hemodynamically significant in less than 50% of cases.[9] The moderate PPV for CTA has remained a challenge and had led to multiple efforts to augment the anatomic information provided by CTA. Although computed tomography perfusion imaging has shown the potential to improve the PPV, this approach significantly complicates image acquisition and lengthens the time a patient would need to be on the CT scanner, while increasing contrast dose and radiation exposure for the patient. Coronary computed tomography

fractional flow reserve (CT-FFR) has emerged as a disruptive technology that offers insight into the hemodynamic consequence of a specific anatomic coronary lesion. The CT-FFR technique uses the CTA images and computational fluid dynamic (CFD) techniques to estimate virtual FFR values throughout the coronary tree (**Fig. 1**).[12] Several multicenter trials have demonstrated that CT-FFR has a significantly higher predictive value for functionally obstructive lesions as defined by invasive FFR, and the technique is poised to become a potential gate-keeper to the catheterization laboratory. This article reviews the hemodynamic concepts and methodology for performing FFR and CT-FFR and reviews the diagnostic and prognostic information from CT-FFR that can be used to guide coronary interventions.

INVASIVE ASSESSMENT OF FRACTIONAL FLOW RESERVE

In 1974, Gould and colleagues[13] performed a landmark canine study using Technetium-99, a gamma camera, and sodium diatrizoate as a hyperemic agent, demonstrating that although resting perfusion was normal in the setting of a left circumflex (LCX) coronary artery occlusion, perfusion in the LCX territory in the presence of maximal hyperemia was significantly reduced.[14] Therefore, vasodilator stress testing led to the subsequent proliferation of myocardial perfusion imaging to noninvasively assess for obstructive CAD. In 1984, White and colleagues[15] used an intracoronary Doppler flow wire to invasively measure coronary flow reserve (CFR) to determine the functional severity of lesions within a given coronary artery; the investigators demonstrated that visual assessment resulted in the significant overestimation of lesion severity. In the early 1990s, studies[16-18] revealed that relative CFR, which has become known as FFR, correlated with significant epicardial stenosis and was less impacted by other physiologic factors, such as heart rate and blood pressure, compared with CFR.

FFR is defined as the ratio of the flow through a coronary stenosis (Q_s) to the flow in the coronary artery in the absence of a coronary stenosis (Q_n). By applying Poiseuille's law, the fluid dynamic equivalent of Ohm's law, the laminar blood flow within a vessel (Q) can be equated to the driving pressure (ΔP) divided by the resistance (R). Under the assumption of minimal contribution of collateral flow, and assuming that in the setting of maximal hyperemia the venous pressure (Pv) is much lower than the pressure distal

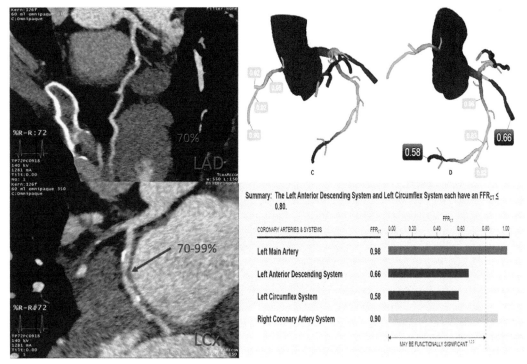

Fig. 1. (*Left*) FFR-CT performed using HeartFlow shows hemodynamically significant lesions in the identified arteries. (*Right*) CT images show greater than 70% lesions (*arrow*) in both left anterior descending (LAD) and LCX arteries.

to the stenosis (*Pd*) and the arterial pressure (*Pa*) upstream of the stenosis, the expression for FFR is equivalent to the ratio of *Pd* to *Pa*, or:

$$\text{FFR} = \frac{Qs}{Qn} = \frac{Pd}{Pa} \qquad (1)$$

The development of catheters with highly accurate pressure transducers has made it possible to simultaneously measure *Pa* and *Pd* in a state of hyperemia with a high degree of fidelity (**Fig. 2**). This approach of using the ratio of *Pd* to *Pa* in a state of hyperemia to calculate FFR was initially validated in a cohort of 45 consecutive patients with moderate coronary stenosis and chest pain who underwent concomitant stress testing.[19] Reversible myocardial ischemia, as defined by the combination of noninvasive stress tests, was identified in all 21 patients with an FFR less than 0.75, resulting in a sensitivity of 88%, a specificity of 100%, and an accuracy of 93% for FFR.[19] Furthermore, a meta-analysis correlating invasive FFR to noninvasive imaging showed a sensitivity and specificity of 76%.[20] Reproducibility of invasive FFR is also excellent with standard deviation of 0.018 and coefficient of variation of 2.5%.[21] FFR is a viable measure of significant epicardial stenosis and a possible application in certain clinical settings.[22,23]

COMPUTER TOMOGRAPHY FRACTIONAL FLOW RESERVE

In the setting of stable ischemic heart disease, guidelines recommend the use of noninvasive functional imaging before ICA or invasive assessment of FFR to determine the functional significance of a coronary stenosis. Although coronary CTA provides an excellent visual assessment of a stenotic lesion by its anatomic nature, it has limited specificity for predicting the hemodynamic significance of coronary stenosis as defined by invasive FFR.

To overcome this limitation, CT-FFR was developed by Taylor and colleagues[12] using the conceptual framework of FFR and advanced computational modeling. This technique enables an approximation of FFR from standard coronary CTA images without additional imaging or medications. CTA FFR requires the creation of an anatomic model of the coronary vasculature, a mathematical model of coronary physiology, and a computational model of the fluid dynamics (**Fig. 3**). A patient-specific anatomic model of the aortic root and epicardial coronary arteries is generated from the CTA data using semiautomatic coronary segmentation algorithms. As resting coronary blood flow is proportional to the left ventricular mass downstream of the vessel of interest, resting coronary blood flow can be estimated using allometric scaling laws and an assessment of

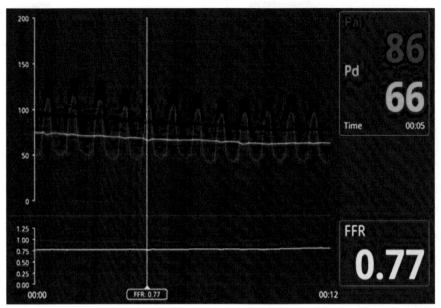

Fig. 2. An example of invasive FFR with use of adenosine in a patient with angiographically intermediate lesion but hemodynamically significant by FFR.

myocardial mass derived from coronary CTA data. Cardiac output is similarly computed using allometric scaling laws and a patient's mean aortic pressure, which is estimated from a patient's measured mean brachial pressure. The Navier-Stokes equations, which describe the flow of viscous fluids, are solved numerically using CFD techniques that use anatomic data and boundary conditions, representing cardiac output, aortic pressure, and microcirculatory resistance. Maximal hyperemia is simulated by reducing the peripheral resistance by a factor of 0.24, approximating the

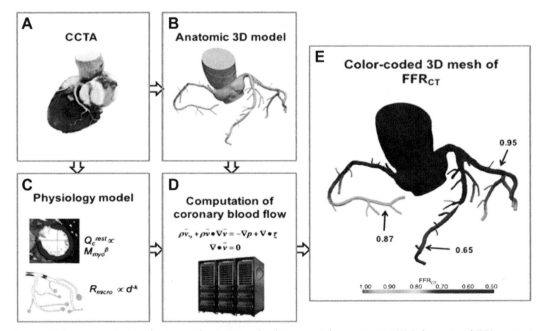

Fig. 3. (*A*) Coronary commuted tomography angiography data are used to generate a (*B*) 3-dimensional (3D) anatomic model. (*C*) Patient-specific physiologic model of microcirculation is created. (*D*) CFD is used to compute coronary blood flow. (*E*) CT-FFR is calculated at each location in the coronary tree. (*Adapted from* Nørgaard BL, Leipsic J, Gaur S, et al. Diagnostic performance of noninvasive fractional flow reserve derived from coronary computed tomography angiography in suspected coronary artery disease: the NXT trial. J Am Coll Cardiol 2014;63(12):1148; with permission.)

effect of 140 μg/kg/min of adenosine typically used for pharmacologic stress testing. From this simulation of blood flow under hyperemic conditions, FFR can be determined by solving for the velocity and pressure distribution within the coronary vessel and proximal aorta. The ratio of computed pressure distal to the lesion of interest in the specific coronary vessel and pressure in the aorta under hyperemic conditions is then used as a surrogate of the invasively derived FFR.[12] Currently, HeartFlow (Redwood City, CA, USA) has the only US Food and Drug Administration–approved process for the clinical determination of CT-FFR. The process involves uploading the CTA data to HeartFlow's servers, where the segmentation is performed and CFD are computed; then the coronary tree showing the distribution of CT-FFR throughout the tree is sent back to the provider. Currently, the turnaround time is less than 14 hours in most cases, and the company is aiming for a 1-hour turnaround time in the future.

Because of the high computational demand of CFD, machine-learning approaches are being developed as an alternative approach with the potential for "on-site" rapid evaluation of CT-FFR. In developing this neural-network model, blood flow computations derived from CFDs are simulated in 12,000 unique, realistic, synthetically generated coronary anatomies.[24] These data are then used to train a deep learning framework that calculates machine learning based coronary fractional flow reserve ($cFFR_{ML}$). Once the model is trained, $cFFR_{ML}$ can be determined at each segment of the coronary anatomy. Furthermore, this can be accomplished in seconds instead of hours because it only involves applying the machine-learning network to the data, rather than complex, time-consuming computations.[24]

To validate the machine-learning approach, trained models were compared with CFD in a study of 87 patients, 125 lesions in total.[24] The correlation between these 2 approaches was 0.9994 ($P<.001$).[24] In this same study, the machine-learning approach was compared with invasive FFR, and a total of 38 of the 125 lesions were found to have a hemodynamically significant lesion using the invasive method, defined as an FFR ≤ 0.80. With this as the gold standard, machine-learning–based FFR had a sensitivity of 81%, a specificity of 84%, and an accuracy of 83%. The correlation was relatively strong as well, at 0.729 ($P<.001$).[24]

DIAGNOSTIC PERFORMANCE OF COMPUTED TOMOGRAPHY-FRACTIONAL FLOW RESERVE

As described above, there are 2 primary approaches to CT-FFR that have been evaluated clinically. The commercial product developed by HeartFlow has been used in most clinical validation studies, with a smaller number of studies using $cFFR_{ML}$, which is currently used in research and not clinically available.

The DISCOVER-FLOW trial was a prospective multicenter study of 103 patients with suspected or known CAD undergoing CTA, ICA, and invasive FFR.[25] Per imaged vessel, the accuracy, sensitivity, and specificity were 58.5%, 91.4%, and 39.6%, respectively, for CTA versus 84.3%, 87.9%, and 82.2%, respectively, for CT-FFR.[25] There was a significant improvement in specificity and accuracy with the use of CT-FFR over CTA alone (**Fig. 4**). The DeFACTO trial was a prospective multicenter study of 252 stable patients with known or suspected CAD. Patients underwent

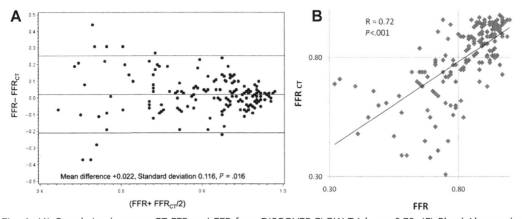

Fig. 4. (A) Correlation between CT-FFR and FFR from DISCOVER-FLOW Trial, r = 0.72. (B) Bland-Altman plot showing slight underestimation of CT-FFR and observed FFR. (*From* Koo BK, Erglis A, Doh JH, et al. Diagnosis of ischemia-causing coronary stenoses by noninvasive fractional flow reserve computed from coronary computed tomographic angiograms. J Am Coll Cardiol 2011;58:1995; with permission.)

CTA, CT-FFR, ICA, and invasive FFR.[26] On a per-patient basis, the sensitivity, specificity, and accuracy were 84%, 42%, and 64%, respectively, for coronary CTA and were 90%, 54%, and 73%, respectively, for CT-FFR.[26] In this study, roughly 11% of cases had insufficient image quality for assessment of CT-FFR.[27] Like DISCOVER-FLOW, DeFACTO showed an improvement in specificity of CT-FFR compared with CTA alone; in addition, it also showed evidence of improved discriminatory power with an area under the curve (AUC) of 0.81 for CT-FFR compared with 0.61 for CTA alone (P<.001).[26] However, this study did not meet its primary endpoint of improved accuracy compared with coronary CTA. The NXT trial was a prospective multicenter study of 254 patients scheduled to undergo coronary angiography.[11] NXT used an improved CT-FFR algorithm and had more stringent CTA imaging protocols. On a per-patient basis, the sensitivity, specificity, and accuracy of CTA was 94%, 34%, and 53%, respectively, and was 88%, 79%, and 81%, respectively, for CT-FFR.[11]

Several meta-analyses of the performance of CT-FFR have been performed. Gonzalez and colleagues[10] pooled data from 18 studies that compared either CTA or CT-FFR to invasive FFR. Although the pooled sensitivities of CT-FFR and CTA were comparable, CT-FFR had a higher per-patient specificity of 77% as compared with that of CT, which had a specificity of only 43% (Fig. 5). A recent meta-analysis by Cook and colleagues[28] pooled data from 5 studies that compared CT-FFR to invasive FFR (cutoff 0.8) and found an overall accuracy of

CT-FFR of 82% at a CT-FFR cutoff of 0.8. For lesions with a CT-FFR greater than 0.9, there was a 97.8% chance that the invasive FFR was greater than 0.8, indicating the absence of ischemia, whereas for lesions with a CT-FFR less than 0.6, there was 87.5% certainty that the invasive FFR was less than 0.8, indicating ischemia. However, in the CT-FFR range of 0.6 to 0.9, near the critical invasive FFR cut point of 0.8, the agreement was significantly poorer.

Several studies have assessed the diagnostic accuracy of "on-site" CT-FFR_ML. Yang and colleagues[29] analyzed 72 patients with invasive FFR from a prospective stress CT myocardial perfusion registry. CT-FFR values were determined from the rest phase of the CT perfusion studies and demonstrated sensitivities and specificities of 87% and 77% for CT-FFR_ML, respectively, as compared with 94% and 66% for CTA alone.[29] There was also a significantly higher AUC (0.913 for CT-FFR vs 0.856 for CTA, P = .004).[29] In a separate study comparing "on-site" evaluation of CT-FFR_ML and CT perfusion on 74 patients,[30] there was a significant improvement in specificity and accuracy of 60% versus 49% and 70% versus 63%, respectively, when comparing CT-FFR versus CTA alone.[30] A recently published meta-analysis pooled data from 8 total studies, including the "on-site" studies previously discussed, showed a pooled sensitivity and specificity of 93% and 82%, respectively.[27] Diagnostic accuracy was near 90% if the CT-FFR range was restricted to less than 0.74 because it has been shown that intermediate stenosis and calcifications can limit diagnostic accuracy.[27]

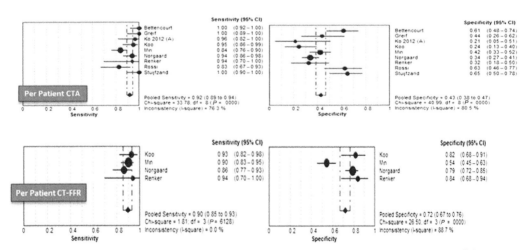

Fig. 5. Meta-analysis showing significant improvement in specificity with per patient CT-FFR. CI, confidence interval; df, degrees of freedom. (Adapted from Gonzalez JA, Lipinski MJ, Flors L, et al. Meta-analysis of diagnostic performance of coronary computed tomography angiography, computed tomography perfusion, and computed tomography-fractional flow reserve in functional myocardial ischemia assessment versus invasive fractional flow reserve. Am J Cardiol 2015;116(9):1472; with permission.)

USING COMPUTED TOMOGRAPHY-FRACTIONAL FLOW RESERVE TO GUIDE CLINICAL MANAGEMENT

Several recent studies have looked at whether the addition of CT-FFR to traditional risk stratification pathways impacts clinical management. In 2015, the PLATFORM trial was the first to study clinical outcomes with the use of CT-FFR compared with "usual care."[31] The study enrolled 584 symptomatic patients without known CAD with a planned noninvasive evaluation or planned ICA. In the planned noninvasive test group, patients were randomized to their standard noninvasive test versus CTA with CT-FFR. In the planned invasive group, patients were randomized to ICA versus CTA with CT-FFR.[31] In patients referred for noninvasive testing, there was no difference between "usual care" and CT-FFR–guided therapy in clinical events at 3 months. However, for patients initially referred for ICA, there were significantly lower rates of nonobstructive CAD in the CT-FFR group.[31] Cost analysis data from PLATFORM showed a 32% reduction in mean costs in the FFR-CT group compared with the "usual care" group for the planned invasive patients.[32] Costs were not different between CT-FFR and "usual care" in the noninvasive group; however, a clear benefit in quality-of-life scores was seen in this group.[32]

The PROMISE trial was an observational cohort study of stable chest pain patients randomized to an anatomic (CTA) versus functional analysis that demonstrated similar outcomes for either evaluation strategy. In a post hoc analysis, CT-FFR was performed in patients in the CTA arm who underwent ICA within 90 days.[33] As the CT-FFR was performed after the completion of the trial, the impact on coronary evaluation and treatment could not be directly assessed. Interestingly, a CT-FFR of less than 0.81 was a better predictor of revascularization and major adverse cardiac events (MACE) compared with severe CTA stenosis (hazard ratio of 4.3 vs 2.9; $P = .033$).[33] The investigators concluded that the use of CT-FFR and an FFR less than 0.81 could decrease the need for ICA by 44%.[33] The CT-FFR RIPCORD Study asked the question, "Does routine availability of CT-derived FFR influence management of the patient with stable chest pain compared with CTA alone?"[34] The study enrolled 200 stable chest pain patients who underwent CTA and CT-FFR. Clinical management was made by consensus from 3 experienced interventional cardiologists based on CTA results alone. Then, CT-FFR results were revealed, and another plan was determined by the same interventional cardiologists. A change in clinical management occurred in 72 cases or 36%.[34] The main factor driving the change in management was a CT-FFR calculated as greater than 0.8 in 13 of 44 vessels (29.5%) that were graded as greater than 90% by CTA alone.[34] In Denmark, a real world evaluation of CT-FFR was performed at Aarhus University. The investigators reviewed the complete diagnostic workup of 1248 nonemergent patients referred for coronary CTA.[35] CT-FFR was performed on 189 patients, and 31% were found to have a CT-FFR of ≤0.80.[35] Of those patients, 29% were referred for ICA, and invasive FFR was measured in 19% with another 1% having instantaneous free wave ratio (iFR) performed.[35] CT-FFR of ≤0.80 correctly identified 73% of patient with an invasive FFR ≤0.8 or iFR ≤0.9.[35] The accuracy of detecting an abnormal invasive FFR was only 50% for CT-FFR in the range of 0.76 to 0.8, whereas it was 75% in the range of 0.71 to 0.75, and 100% for CT-FFR less than 0.7. Therefore, a lower cutoff for CT-FFR such as less than 0.75 may have greater accuracy with respect to invasive FFR. Of note, there were no adverse cardiac events seen in patients who had a calculated CT-FFR greater than 0.80.[35]

In summary, several studies now suggest that CT-FFR could lead to the reduction of unnecessary ICA in patients who are likely to have nonobstructive CAD.[31,32,34] Despite ICA having a low risk of major adverse events, the risks of bleeding, contrast, radiation, and major vascular injury do exist, and it would be best to prevent unneeded ICA if possible. Per the PLATFORM study, there may also be a cost savings to a CT-FFR strategy, particularly in patients with stable chest pain referred for an invasive strategy, along with improvement in the patient's perception of chest pain in the noninvasive strategy arm.[32]

LIMITATIONS OF COMPUTED TOMOGRAPHY-FRACTIONAL FLOW RESERVE

Based on current studies, CT-FFR has primarily been validated against FFR in relatively low-risk patients. Thus, the understanding of the performance of CT-FFR in intermediate-risk patients remains limited.[28] In addition, there are some limitations to the technology itself. First, it is based on a proprietary algorithm, and access to the technology is currently limited. However, adoption of payment for CT-FFR by payers will likely broaden the clinical availability of CT-FFR. In addition, image quality is of particular importance.[26] In trials including DISCOVER-FLOW, NXT, and DeFACTO, CTA data required an independent review from HeartFlow to determine suitability of CT-FFR analysis. In these studies, the number of rejected datasets ranged from 11% to 13%.[11,25,27] In the PROMISE analysis, 33% of studies sent to the core laboratory were rejected as inadequate for CT-FFR analysis. This population only included patients that underwent ICA in the PROMISE trial, and thus, the cases referred to ICA may have had poorer CTA quality. In a single-center review in a highly experienced center, 10% to 15% of cases that were referred for CT-FFR were rejected because of inadequate image quality.[35] Because the boundary conditions for the CFD are derived from the coronary anatomy from CTA, issues such as significant coronary calcifications could limit the quality of the anatomic models.[36] One study, however, has demonstrated similar performance of CT-FFR in the presence or absence of coronary calcifications.[37] Currently, CT-FFR cannot assess lesions with myocardial stents or bypass grafts.

FUTURE APPLICATIONS AND POTENTIAL FOR COMPUTED TOMOGRAPHY-FRACTIONAL FLOW RESERVE

Although CT-FFR is becoming a mature technology, it remains an active area of technical and clinical research. There is significant interest in using machine-learning techniques to improve analysis times, which could broaden the clinical applicability, particularly in the setting of acute chest pain.[38,39] Several studies are looking at the role of CT-FFR in evaluation of acute chest pain in the emergency room, where CTA has been shown to reduce evaluation time and unnecessary hospitalizations.[40]

CT-FFR may also be useful for planning of complex interventions where "virtual stenting" can be used to predict the hemodynamic effect of coronary stenting.[41] A study of 44 prospectively enrolled patients showed that the diagnostic accuracy of CT-FFR measurement after virtual stenting as compared with invasive FFR following actual stenting was 96%.[42] There could also be a benefit in the assessment of serial stenosis, which can be a challenge with invasive FFR.[43] The clinical impact of virtual stenting has yet to be evaluated. Currently, CT-FFR cannot be performed in coronary artery vein grafts. Further studies are needed to assess the impact of collateralization on noninvasively measured CT-FFR, in addition to assess whether CT-FFR can play a role in vein grafts.

The combination of CT-FFR and CT perfusion has shown promise for further improving the accuracy of CTA in the evaluation of stable chest pain.[30] Several ongoing clinical trials, such as NCT02208388, are actively enrolling patients to assess whether the combination of CT perfusion and CT-FFR will be useful to guide therapy. Currently, the clinical impact of the combination of CT perfusion and CT-FFR is unknown.

SUMMARY

Although CTA has high sensitivity and NPV for excluding functionally significant CAD as defined by invasive FFR, its moderate specificity and PPV have remained a significant limitation. CT-FFR can significantly improve the specificity and PPV of CTA, potentially broadening the clinical utility of a coronary CTA evaluation strategy. There is growing evidence demonstrating improvement in important outcomes, such as reducing the need for invasive procedures, improving quality of life, and reducing health care costs. The application of deep learning to CT-FFR analysis has the potential to reduce computational times leading to broader applicability of CT-FFR. CT-FFR has demonstrated significant promise as a noninvasive technique to evaluate the functional severity of coronary stenosis, which has the potential for significant cost savings by serving as a gate-keeper for ICA.

REFERENCES

1. Tonino PA, De Bruyne B, Pijls NH, et al. Fractional flow reserve versus angiography for guiding percutaneous coronary intervention. N Engl J Med 2009; 360:213–24.
2. Tonino PA. Angiographic versus functional severity of coronary artery stenosis in the FAME study fractional flow reserve versus angiography in multivessel evaluation. J Am Coll Cardiol 2010;55:2816–21.
3. Pijls NH, Fearon WF, Tonino PA, et al. Fractional flow reserve versus angiography for guiding percutaneous coronary intervention in patients with multivessel coronary artery disease: 2-year follow-up of the FAME (Fractional Flow Reserve Versus Angiography for Multivessel Evaluation) study. J Am Coll Cardiol 2010;56(3):177–84.
4. van Nunen LX, Zimmermann FM, Tonino PA, et al. Fractional flow reserve versus angiography for guidance of PCI in patients with multivessel coronary artery disease (FAME): 5-year follow-up of a randomised controlled trial. Lancet 2015; 386(10006):1853–60.
5. De Bruyne B, Pijls NH, Kalesan B, et al. Fractional flow reserve-guided PCI versus medical therapy in

stable coronary disease. N Engl J Med 2012; 367(11):991–1001.

6. Fihn SD, Blankenship JC, Alexander KP, et al. 2014 ACC/AHA/AATS/PCNA/SCAI/STS Focused update of the guideline for the diagnosis and management of patients with stable ischemic heart disease: a report of the American College of Cardiology/ American Heart Association Task Force on Practice Guidelines, and the American Association for Thoracic Surgery, Preventive Cardiovascular Nurses Association, Society for Cardiovascular Angiography and Interventions, and Society of Thoracic Surgeons. J Am Coll Cardiol 2014;64(18):1929–49.

7. Patel MR, Calhoon J, Dehmer GJ, et al. ACC/AATS/ AHA/ASE/ASNC/SCAI/SCCT/STS 2017 Appropriate use criteria for coronary revascularization in patients with stable ischemic heart disease : a report of the American College of Cardiology Appropriate Use Criteria Task Force, American Association for Thoracic Surgery, American Heart Association, American Society of Echocardiography, American Society of Nuclear Cardiology, Society for Cardiovascular Angiography and Interventions, Society of Cardiovascular Computed Tomography, and Society of Thoracic Surgeons. J Nucl Cardiol 2017; 24(5):1759–92.

8. Patel MR, Peterson ED, David D, et al. Low diagnostic yield of elective coronary angiography. N Engl J Med 2010;362:886–95.

9. Meijboom WB, Van Mieghem CA, van Pelt N, et al. Comprehensive assessment of coronary artery stenoses: computed tomography coronary angiography versus conventional coronary angiography and correlation with fractional flow reserve in patients with stable angina. J Am Coll Cardiol 2008; 52:636–43.

10. Gonzalez JA, Lipinski MJ, Flors L, et al. Meta-analysis of diagnostic performance of coronary computed tomography angiography, computed tomography perfusion, and computed tomography-fractional flow reserve in functional myocardial ischemia assessment versus invasive fractional flow reserve. Am J Cardiol 2015;116(9):1469–78.

11. Nørgaard BL, Leipsic J, Gaur S, et al. Diagnostic performance of noninvasive fractional flow reserve derived from coronary computed tomography angiography in suspected coronary artery disease: the NXT trial (analysis of coronary blood flow using CT angiography: next steps). J Am Coll Cardiol 2014;63(12):1145–55.

12. Taylor CA, Fonte TA, Min JK. Computational fluid dynamics applied to cardiac computed tomography for noninvasive quantification of fractional flow reserve: scientific basis. J Am Coll Cardiol 2013;61(22):2233–41.

13. Gould KL, Lipscomb K, Hamilton GW. Physiologic basis for assessing critical coronary stenosis: instantaneous flow response and regional distribution during coronary hyperemia as measures of coronary flow reserve. Am J Card 1974;33(1):87–94.

14. Kirkeeide RL, Gould KL, Parsel L. Assessment of coronary stenoses by myocardial perfusion imaging during pharmacologic coronary vasodilation. VII. Validation of coronary flow reserve as a single integrated functional measure of stenosis severity reflecting all its geometric dimensions. J Am Coll Cardiol 1986;7:103–13.

15. White CW, Wright CB, Doty DB, et al. Does visual interpretation of the coronary arteriogram predict the physiological importance of a coronary stenosis. N Engl J Med 1984;310:819–24.

16. Gould KL, Kirkeeide RL, Buchi M. Coronary flow reserve as a physiologic measure of stenosis severity. J Am Coll Cardiol 1990;15:459–74.

17. Pijls NH, van Son JA, Kirkeeide RL, et al. Experimental basis of determining maximum coronary, myocardial, and collateral blood flow by pressure measurements for assessing functional stenosis severity before and after percutaneous transluminal coronary angioplasty. Circulation 1993;87:1354–67.

18. Johnson NP, Kirkeeide RL, Gould KL. History and development of coronary flow reserve and fractional flow reserve for clinical applications. Interv Cardiol Clin 2015;4(4):397–410.

19. Pijls NH, De Bruyne B, Peels K, et al. Measurement of fractional flow reserve to assess the functional severity of coronary-artery stenosis. N Engl J Med 1996;334:1703–8.

20. Christou MA, Siontis GC, Katritsis DG, et al. Meta-analysis of fractional flow reserve versus quantitative coronary angiography and noninvasive imaging for evaluation of myocardial ischemia. Am J Cardiol 2007;99:450–6.

21. Johnson NP, Johnson DT, Kirkeeide RL, et al. Repeatability of fractional flow reserve despite variations in systemic and coronary hemodynamics. JACC Cardiovasc Intv 2015;8:1018–27.

22. De Bruyne B, Pijls NH, Bartunek J, et al. Fractional flow reserve in patients with prior myocardial infarction. Circulation 2001;104:157–62.

23. Pijls NH, Van Gelder B, Van der Voort P, et al. Fractional flow reserve: a useful index to evaluate the influence of an epicardial coronary stenosis on myocardial blood flow. Circulation 1995;92: 3183–93.

24. Itu L, Rapaka A, Passerini T, et al. A machine learning approach for computation of fractional flow reserve from coronary computed tomography. J Appl Physiol (1985) 2016;121(1):42–52.

25. Koo BK, Erglis A, Doh JH, et al. Diagnosis of ischemia-causing coronary stenoses by noninvasive fractional flow reserve computed from coronary computed tomographic angiograms. J Am Coll Cardiol 2011;58:1989–97.

26. Nakazato R, Park HB, Berman DS, et al. Noninvasive fractional flow reserve derived from computed tomography angiography for coronary lesions of intermediate stenosis severity: results from the DeFACTO study. Circ Cardiovasc Imaging 2013; 6(6):881–9.

27. Tesche C, De Cecco CN, Albrecht MH, et al. Coronary CT angiography-derived fractional flow reserve. Radiology 2017;285(1):17–33.

28. Cook CM, Petraco R, Shun-Shin MJ, et al. Diagnostic accuracy of computed tomography-derived fractional flow reserve: a systematic review. JAMA Cardiol 2017;2(7):803–10.

29. Yang DR, Kim YH, Roh JH, et al. Diagnostic performance of on-site CT-derived fractional flow reserve versus CT perfusion. Eur Heart J Cardiovasc Imaging 2017;18:432–40.

30. Coenen A, Rossi A, Lubbers MM, et al. Integrating CT myocardial perfusion and CT-FFR in the work-up of coronary artery disease. JACC Cardiovasc Imaging 2017;10:760–70.

31. Douglas PS, Pontone G, Hlatky MA, et al. Clinical outcomes of fractional flow reserve by computed tomographic angiography-guided diagnostic strategies vs usual care in patients with suspected coronary artery disease: the prospective longitudinal trial of FFR(CT): outcome and resource impacts study. Eur Heart J 2015;36(47):3359–67.

32. Hlatky MA, Bruyne BD, Pontone G, et al. Quality-of-life and economic outcomes of assessing fractional flow reserve with computed tomography angiography: PLATFORM. J Am Coll Cardiol 2015;66:2315–23.

33. Lu MT, Ferencik M, Roberts RS, et al. Noninvasive FFR derived from coronary CT angiography: management and outcomes in the PROMISE trial. JACC Cardiovasc Imaging 2017;10(11):1350–8.

34. Curzen NP, Nolan J, Zaman AG, et al. Does the routine availability of CT-derived FFR influence management of patients with stable chest pain compared to ct angiography alone?: The FFRCT RIPCORD study. JACC Cardiovasc Imaging 2016; 9:1188–94.

35. Nørgaard BL, Hjort J, Gaur S, et al. Clinical use of coronary CTA–derived FFR for decision-making in stable CAD. JACC Cardiovasc Imaging 2017;10: 541–50.

36. Nørgaard BL, Leipsic J, Bon-Kown K, et al. Coronary computed tomography angiography derived fractional flow reserve and plaque stress. Curr Cardiovasc Imaging Rep 2016;9:2.

37. Nørgaard BL, Gaur S, Leipsic J, et al. Influence of coronary calcification on the diagnostic performance of CT angiography derived FFR in coronary artery disease: a substudy of the NXT trial. JACC Cardiovasc Imaging 2015;8(9):1045–55.

38. Giannopoulos A, Tang A, Ge Y, et al. Diagnostic performance of a lattice Boltzmann-based method for fast CT-fractional flow reserve. EuroIntervention 2018;13(14):1696–704.

39. Zreik M, Lessmann N, van Hamersvelt RW, et al. Deep learning analysis of the myocardium in coronary CT angiography for identification of patients with functionally significant coronary artery stenosis. Med Image Anal 2017;44:72–85.

40. Hoffman U, Truong QA, Schoenfeld DA, et al. Coronary CT angiography versus standard evaluation in acute chest pain. N Engl J Med 2012;367: 299–308.

41. Morris PD, Ryan D, Morton AC, et al. Virtual fractional flow reserve from coronary angiography: modeling the significance of coronary lesions: results from the VIRTU-1 (VIRTUal Fractional Flow Reserve From Coronary Angiography) study. JACC cardiovasc Interv 2013;6(2):149–57.

42. Kim KH, Doh JH, Koo BK, et al. A novel noninvasive technology for treatment planning using virtual coronary stenting and computed tomography-derived computed fractional flow reserve. JACC Cardiovasc Interv 2014;7:72–8.

43. Ihdayhid AR, White A, Brian KO. Assessment of serial coronary stenosis with noninvasive computed tomography-derived fractional flow reserve and treatment planning using novel virtual stenting application. JACC Cardiovasc Interv 2017;10(24):223–5.

Myocardial Viability Testing to Guide Coronary Revascularization

Adrián I. Löffler, MD[a], Christopher M. Kramer, MD[a,b],*

KEYWORDS

• Viability • Hibernation • Revascularization • Chronic total occlusion

KEY POINTS

- Left ventricular dysfunction remains one of the best prognostic determinants of survival in patients with coronary artery disease and revascularization improves survival.
- Patients with myocardial viability have increased mortality if treated medically and do not undergo revascularization.
- Out of the most commonly used modalities to assess viability, CMR and PET offer the highest sensitivity and specificity.
- Patients undergoing CMR-guided CTO intervention have been shown to have improvement in LV ejection fraction, myocardial perfusion reserve, and symptoms.

INTRODUCTION

Left ventricular (LV) dysfunction remains one of the best prognostic determinants of survival in patients with coronary artery disease (CAD).[1,2] It was originally thought that dysfunctional myocardium after an infarction was irreversibly damaged.[3] However, it was later recognized that some of the involved tissue remained viable and contractility may be restored with revascularization.[4,5] Given that worsening LV systolic function secondary to ischemia has been shown to be associated with worse outcomes, but not all myocardium improves with revascularization, viability testing has since been well studied and used. This article reviews the pathophysiology and mechanism of myocardial viability, the most commonly used noninvasive modalities to assess myocardial viability and their strengths and weaknesses, the utility of viability testing for chronic total occlusion (CTO) interventions, and the STICH trial.[6]

PATHOPHYSIOLOGY AND MECHANISM OF MYOCARDIAL VIABILITY

After a myocardial infarction, the myocardium usually demonstrates one of five pathophysiologies: (1) normal myocardial perfusion and function, (2) myocardial ischemia, (3) stunned myocardium, (4) myocardial hibernation, and (5) nonviable infarction.[3] Prompt reperfusion or the presence of collateral vessels and intact coronary microvasculature function may preserve myocardial perfusion. Ischemia occurs as a result of decreased blood flow resulting in low ATP production and subsequent LV dysfunction.[3]

Myocardial Stunning

Myocardial stunning is a reversible state of regional contractile dysfunction that occurs after transient ischemia without ensuing necrosis.[7] Myocardial stunning is believed to play an important role in persistent contractile dysfunction seen in patients with acute myocardial

Disclosures: Supported in part by NIH, NIBIB (5T32EB003841).
[a] Division of Cardiovascular Medicine, University of Virginia Health System, Box 800170, 1215 Lee Street, Charlottesville, VA 22908, USA; [b] Department of Radiology and Medical Imaging, Cardiovascular Imaging Center, University of Virginia Health System, Box 800170, 1215 Lee Street, Charlottesville, VA 22908, USA
* Corresponding author. University of Virginia Health System, Box 800170, 1215 Lee Street, Charlottesville, VA 22908.
E-mail address: ckramer@virginia.edu

infarction after successful reperfusion.[8] In general, myocardial perfusion is normal and function recovers quickly.

Myocardial Hibernation

More than 40 years ago physicians noticed that chronic myocardial dysfunction before coronary bypass often improved after revascularization.[4,5] Myocardial hibernation is a state of persistent LV dysfunction that results from chronically reduced blood flow or repetitive stunning without infarction and necrosis. A downregulation in contractile function at rest is thought to represent a protective mechanism to reduce myocardial oxygen requirements and ensure myocyte survival. When severe cellular hypoperfusion and damage occurs, only cellular function that is essential for survival, such as membrane integrity, is preserved. Preserved or increased myocardial glucose metabolism also occurs during this state.

Nonviable Myocardium

If myocardial perfusion is not restored, irreversible myocardial necrosis can occur. The goal of viability testing, detailed in the next section, is to determine if a large portion of dysfunctional myocardium is nonviable in which case the risks would likely outweigh benefit of revascularization.

VIABILITY AND NONINVASIVE IMAGING METHODS OF ASSESSMENT

Viability testing can predict improvement of heart failure symptoms and exercise capacity after revascularization.[9,10] The ability to distinguish viable from nonviable myocardium that is able to recover contractile function following revascularization presents a clinical challenge in current practice.[11] Furthermore, viability testing can have a lower specificity because not all patients with viable myocardium improve function after revascularization.[12]

Medical therapy with revascularization in patients with ischemic cardiomyopathy has been shown to decrease mortality compared with medical therapy alone.[13] The probability of reversing LV remodeling and improving LV systolic function with medical therapy and/or revascularization has been shown to be greater with increased proportions of viable myocardium on noninvasive imaging.[14,15] As shown in Fig. 1, Allman and colleagues[16] demonstrated in a meta-analysis of mostly observational studies that patients with viability treated by revascularization had a near 80% reduction in mortality. Those without

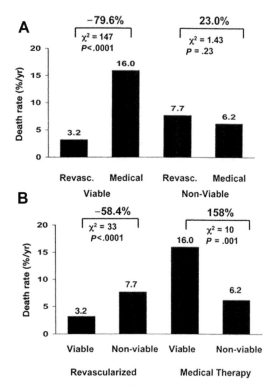

Fig. 1. (A) Death rates for patients with and without myocardial viability treated by revascularization or medical therapy. (B) Same data as A with comparisons based on treatment strategy in patients with and without viability. (From Allman KC, Shaw LJ, Hachamovitch R, et al. Myocardial viability testing and impact of revascularization on prognosis in patients with coronary artery disease and left ventricular dysfunction: a meta-analysis. J Am Coll Cardiol 2002;39(7):1155; with permission.)

viability had no difference in mortality between medical therapy or revascularization. We will next review each of the currently most commonly used modalities for viability testing.

Single-Photon Emission Computed Tomography

Single-photon emission computed tomography (SPECT) uses radionuclide-labeled tracer to measure regional tracer concentration in the myocardium and can measure viability by determining percentage of peak uptake of the tracer. This is interpreted with rest images only or with a stress/rest testing protocol. The most commonly used tracers are ^{99m}Tc-sestamibi or ^{201}Tl. The two tracers have been shown to have comparable results in predicting recovery of resting defects.[17] Radiotracers sequester within myocytes with intact cell membrane. Thus, myocardial viability is interpreted as an all-or-none phenomenon because SPECT cannot assess the transmural extent of variability within the LV wall. The advantage of ^{99m}Tc-sestamibi is its much shorter protocol duration with rest imaging occurring approximately 1 hour after tracer administration. ^{201}T viability imaging is based on its redistributive property of ^{201}Tl in the myocardium and thus requires 4-hour and 24-hour delayed imaged to assess viability.[18]

A cutoff of greater than 50% tracer activity is the most commonly used criteria to identify viable myocardium (Fig. 2). When viability is clearly present on rest images, generally no further imaging is necessary to determine viability. It has been shown that the presence of inducible ischemia is of additive value and more predictive of functional recovery than comparable images with similar peak uptake of tracer on rest images but no ischemia.[19] SPECT has been shown to have a mean sensitivity of 84% and mean specificity of 77% in predicting recovery of global LV function after revascularization.[7]

Dobutamine Stress Echocardiography

Assessment for augmentation of contractility, or contractile reserve, in response to dobutamine stress is the basis for the use of dobutamine stress echocardiography (DSE) as a measurement of viability.[20] An initial infusion of dobutamine at 2.5 µg/kg/min, with gradual increase to 5, 7.5, 10, and 20 µg/kg/min, is commonly used.[21] Wall thickness should be assessed on resting images because segments that are thinned ($\leq$0.5 or 0.6 cm) and bright (suggesting advanced fibrosis) rarely recover.[21–23] DSE has higher specificity (mean, 79% vs 59%) but lower sensitivity (mean, 82% vs 86%) in detection of viable myocardium compared with ^{201}Tl rest-redistribution imaging.[21,24] Less scar and greater percentage of viable myocytes are needed to detect contractile reserve by DSE.[25]

Multicenter studies have shown worse outcomes when viable myocardium is identified by DSE and no revascularization is pursued.[26,27] Four distinct responses to dobutamine echo

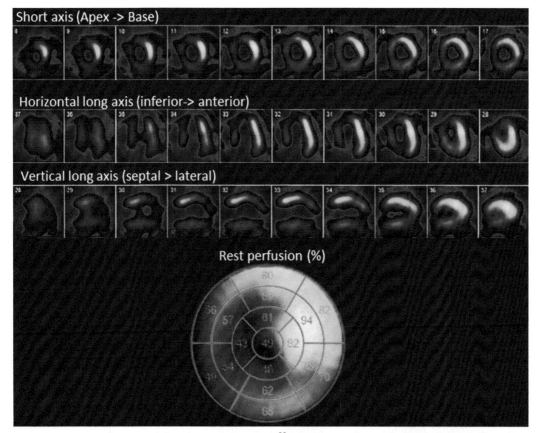

Fig. 2. SPECT rest only myocardial perfusion imaging with ^{99m}Tc-sestamibi for viability assessment of a patient with severe three-vessel disease and LV ejection fraction 35%. Visual and quantitative analysis reveals a large region of infarct in the apical to mid anterior, anteroseptal, and inferoseptal segments. The quantitative polar plot shown reveals viability in all coronary territories except in segments of the apex with perfusion less than 50%.

have been described.[11,21,28] A "biphasic response" can occur in which contractility improves in dysfunctional segments with low-dose dobutamine and then becomes dysfunctional again at higher doses because of ischemia. The biphasic response is 60% sensitive and 88% specific in assessing recovery of contractile function 6 weeks after coronary angioplasty.[28] Another study in patients with ischemic cardiomyopathy undergoing coronary artery bypass graft (CABG) showed a 75% improvement in regional ventricular function after 14 months.[29] Hibernating myocardium is thought to occur with "worsening contractile function" as dobutamine doses increase. Hibernating myocardial tissue has no contractile reserve and increases in demand result in ischemia and further worsens contractility. This response to dobutamine has been shown to be the second most predictive of functional recovery.[28,30] Combining biphasic response with worsening response improves sensitivity to 74% but decreases specificity to 73% in assessing recovery of contractile function.[28] Myocardial stunning is believed to be present when there is "sustained improvement" with increasing dobutamine dose. Finally, lack of viability is believed to be present when there is "no response" to dobutamine, with only 4% of segments recovering after revascularization.[11,29]

Cardiac MRI

Cardiac MRI (CMR) provides information in regards to global LV function and regional wall motion. Viability is assessed using LV end-diastolic wall thickness (EDWT) or response to dobutamine stress similar to DSE as previously described. The most commonly used technique is late gadolinium enhancement (LGE) imaging (Fig. 3). Gadolinium should be avoided in those with advanced renal disease because of the risk of nephrogenic systemic fibrosis, although its incidence has virtually disappeared after adopting guidelines restricting its use.[31,32] Other contraindications to MRI include claustrophobia, certain metallic hardware, and inability to breath hold. Pacemakers and defibrillators are no longer absolute contraindications.[33] Benefits of CMR over DSE and SPECT include excellent spatial imaging and ability to determine transmural variations in viability.

Nearly two decades ago, Kim and colleagues[34] demonstrated that reversibly myocardial dysfunction could be identified by contrast-enhanced CMR before coronary revascularization. Fifty patients with planned revascularization (CABG or percutaneous coronary intervention [PCI]) and regional wall motion abnormalities without unstable angina or New York Heart Association functional class IV heart failure were included in this study. Of the

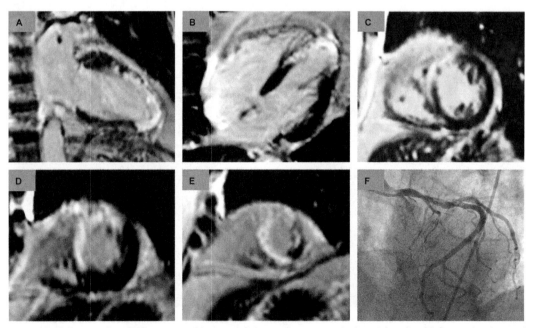

Fig. 3. (A–E) Greater than 75% transmural late gadolinium enhancement in the mid to distal left anterior descending territories suggesting no viability. (F) Coronary angiography demonstrating occluded left anterior descending after late presentation from a myocardial infarct.

patients with dysfunctional segments, 78% of the segments without enhancement (deemed to be completely viable) had an improvement in contractility 79 ± 36 days after revascularization. Reasons for incomplete recovery could be premature reevaluation of ventricular function, tethering to infarcted segments, other nonischemic reasons for LV dysfunction, or incomplete revascularization. Complete recovery of hibernating myocardium may take more than 12 months because prolonged ischemia may result in sarcomere loss, glycogen accumulation, disarray of mitochondria, and fibrosis.[7] A total of 65% of segments with 1% to 25% hyperenhancement and wall segment dysfunction severity of at least severe hypokinesia had recovery in ventricular function after revascularization. A cut-off value of 50% transmural hyperenhancement resulted in a negative predictive value of 92%. An impressive negative predictive accuracy of 100% was seen in segments with at least 75% transmural hyperenhancement and at least severe hypokinesia. LGE CMR has been studied versus PET, the prior gold standard for viability assessment, and found to closely agree in identifying myocardial scar.[35]

A recent meta-analysis by Romero and colleagues[36] studied the three aforementioned CMR methods to assess viability. A cutoff for viability of less than 50% transmural LGE allowed for a high sensitivity (95%) and negative predictive value (90%) but low specificity (51%). Low-dose dobutamine response had the highest specificity (91%) and positive predictive value (93%) with a lower sensitivity (81%) and negative predictive value (75%). Low-dose dobutamine was more accurate than LGE (84% vs 70%). An LV EDWT of 5.5 to 6.0 mm has a high sensitivity (96%) arguing that thin and dysfunctional segments can accurately be classified as nonviable without further assessment with LGE. Specificity, however, is only 38% with this method (Fig. 4).[36] A recent multicenter prospective study using CMR in patients with CAD and regional myocardial thinning found that even in myocardial regions with LV EDWT less than or equal to 5.5 mm an inverse relationship between scar burden (LGE) and viability exist.[37] This suggests that even myocardial segments with regional wall thinning warrant further viability assessment.

PET Imaging with F18-Fluorodeoxyglocse

F-18 Fluorodeoxyglucose (FDG) PET is an effective imaging technique for differentiating among normal, infarcted, stunned, and hibernating myocardium. PET has better spatial resolution than SPECT. Rest perfusion is assessed with multiple tracers, including ^{13}N-ammonia or ^{82}Rb.[38] Hibernating myocardium is determined by assessment of glucose uptake in the myocardium. At rest the myocardium generally oxidizes free fatty acids to produce ATP. However, in the setting of myocardial ischemia, there is a shift to glucose metabolism with up-regulation of glucose transporters. When fasting, FDG is taken up mainly by ischemic myocardium. Scar tissue and normal myocardium do not take up FDG. However, oral glucose loading can stimulate FDG uptake in viable and normal myocardium. Insulin is given to correct for hyperglycemia as needed.[39] In patients with insulin resistance, FDG uptake in normal regions may remain less than that of ischemic or hibernating regions. One limitation to PET is the variability of FDG uptake, which is impacted by cardiac output, heart failure, degree of ischemia, and sympathetic activity.[11]

The typical appearance of hibernation on PET with FDG is a perfusion-metabolism mismatch, which involves decreased ^{13}N-ammonia uptake, indicating decreased perfusion, and increased or preserved FDG uptake caused by up-regulation of glucose transporters.[38] A reduction in blood flow and metabolism is indicative of myocardial scar (Fig. 5). FDG PET can identify stunned myocardium by demonstrating normal perfusion in an area of regional contractile dysfunction.

Tillisch and colleagues[40] demonstrated that FDG PET could predict reversible segments (85% predictive accuracy) and irreversible (92% predictive accuracy) abnormal contraction in patients with LV systolic dysfunction undergoing coronary-artery bypass. Eitzman and colleagues[10] used perfusion and FDG PET to assess viability before revascularization (CABG or PCI) in 82 patients with advanced CAD and LV dysfunction. Those who had evidence of viability who did not undergo revascularization were more likely to experience a myocardial infarction, death, cardiac arrest, or later revascularization (P<.01). Those with viability that underwent revascularization had improvement in symptoms. Those without viability had no difference in outcome comparing revascularization with no revascularization.

A meta-analysis of 20 studies with 598 patients undergoing viability with FDG before revascularization showed a high sensitivity (93%) but low specificity (58%) for identifying LV recovery.[24] Sensitivity was higher than other nuclear imaging techniques and dobutamine echocardiography. The lower specificity was thought to be in part caused by variation of

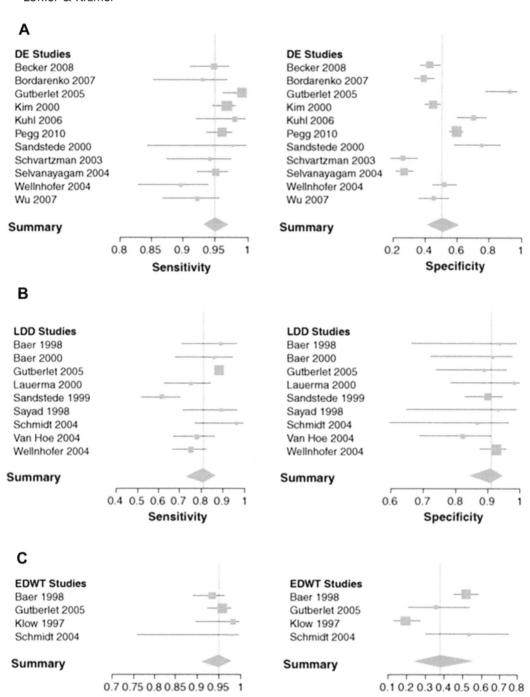

Fig. 4. Forest plots of sensitivity and specificity for (A) delayed enhancement (DE) CMR, (B) low-dose dobutamine (LDD) CMR, and (C) resting LV end-diastolic wall thickness (EDWT). The size of the square plotting symbol is proportional to the same size for each study. Horizontal lines are the 95% confidence intervals, and the summary sensitivity and specificity are calculated based on the bivariate approach. (*From* Romero J, Xue X, Gonzalez W, et al. CMR imaging assessing viability in. patients with chronic ventricular dysfunction due to coronary artery disease: a meta-analysis of prospective trials. JACC Cardiovasc Imaging 2012;5(5):503; with permission.)

follow-up duration with studies varying from 7 days to 14 months.[24]

To date one randomized control trial, the PET and Recovery Following Revascularization-2

(PARR-2) trial, evaluated the efficacy of FDG PET viability imaging in identification of patients with ischemic cardiomyopathy who would benefit most from revascularization.[41] In the FDG PET

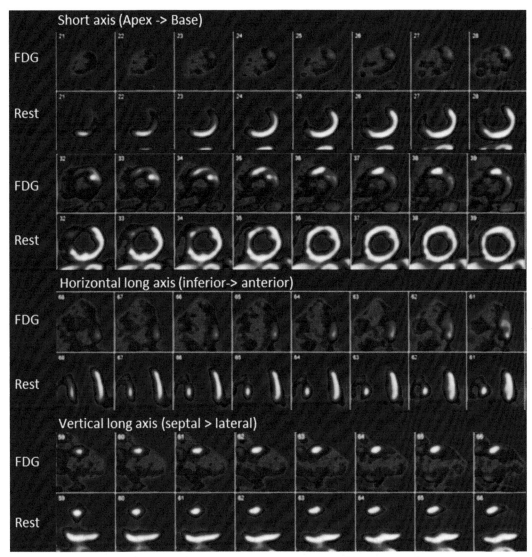

Fig. 5. PET myocardial perfusion imaging using N-13 ammonia rest perfusion images (*bottom row images*) and FDG myocardial metabolic images (*top row images*). A large fixed perfusion defect with akinesis on gated images is seen in the mid to basal anterior and septal segments of the left anterior descending territory. No FDG uptake is seen in this territory suggesting no viability.

assisted management guided arm, when significant viable myocardium was identified revascularization work-up was recommended. When predominantly scar tissue was identified no revascularization work-up was recommended. There was a nonstatistically significant trend ($P = .16$) toward fewer cardiovascular events within 1 year in the FDG-PET assisted management group. A post hoc analysis showed a significant reduction in adverse outcomes ($P = .019$) when there was adherence to PET recommendations. This was a major limitation of the study because only 75% of the patient's clinicians adhered to PET recommendation.[41]

SURGICAL TREATMENT FOR ISCHEMIC HEART FAILURE TRIAL

Surgical Treatment for Ischemic Heart Failure (STICH), was a multicenter, unblinded, randomized control trial evaluating the role of surgical coronary artery revascularization in ischemic cardiomyopathy with ejection fraction (EF) less than or equal to 35%. The main finding was that after a median follow-up of 10 years, surgical revascularization improved all-cause mortality (58.9% vs 66.1%; $P = .02$) and cardiovascular mortality (40.5% vs 49.3%; $P = .006$).[13] A substudy of this trial assessed the 601 patients

Table 1
Pros and cons of each viability modality

Modality	Advantages	Disadvantages
SPECT	• Readily available • Part of routine stress/rest protocol • More sensitive than DSE	• Highest radiation exposure • All-or-none interpretation with inability to assess for hibernation resulting in lower specificity • Prone to attenuation artifacts, especially in obese patients
DSE	• Readily available • No radiation exposure • More specific than SPECT • Can use other predictors of viability, such as LV wall thickness	• Image quality dependent on patient factors (body habitus, lung disease) and experience of sonographer • Lower sensitivity • Contraindicated in patients with tachyarrhythmias and uncontrolled hypertension
CMR	• High-resolution imaging • High sensitivity and specificity • No radiation exposure • Evaluates transmural extent of scar and gold standard for LV volumes and EF assessment • Noncontrast viability methods: dobutamine stress and LV EDWT • Simultaneous evaluation for other etiologies of cardiomyopathy	• Less available • Higher cost • Image quality dependent on electrocardiogram gating and breath-holding • Contraindicated in claustrophobia, certain metal objects, and advanced renal disease for contrast use
PET	• Better spatial resolution, attenuation correction, and diagnostic accuracy than SPECT allowing for better image quality • High sensitivity and specificity • Can differentiate hibernating myocardium from scar	• Less available • Higher cost • Radiation exposure, although less than SPECT • Requires fasting and controlled blood glucose levels

who underwent myocardial viability evaluation with SPECT (n = 321), DSE (n = 130), or both (n = 150) and viability was determined in binary fashion. Mortality was lower in those with viable myocardium (37%) versus without viable myocardium (51%); however, after adjustment for other prognostic variables (age, EF, heart failure class, etc) this association was no longer significant (P = .21). There was also no significant interaction between viability status and treatment assignment with respect to mortality (P = .53).[6]

Some have interpreted these results as viability testing having little value in determining who should undergo revascularization in ischemic cardiomyopathy and as discordance between observational studies with the findings in this trial.[42] However, viability testing in the substudy was not randomized and thus the data were prone to the same biases as an observational study.[43] When this study was initially planned, PET and CMR methods were not available in sufficient numbers of centers to include in the study protocol. Multiple studies have demonstrated superior accuracy of PET and

CMR for assessment of viability compared with T1-201 SPECT and dobutamine echo.[15] One aspect of the trial that could account for its failure to identify benefit from viability testing is that there was a lack of standardized protocols for SPECT viability evaluation. Each center adopted their own SPECT protocol and ischemia assessment was not included. There was also difficulty with patient enrollment, which may be caused by perception of a lack of equipoise among many clinicians. The STICH population also was skewed in that the patients most likely to benefit from CABG may have been selected out either by design or clinician preference.

CHRONIC TOTAL OCCLUSION AND VIABILITY

The benefits of CTO interventions are controversial given the increased complexity of the intervention and the results of the Occluded Artery Trial (OAT), which showed a lack of benefit of PCI versus medical therapy in patients with an occluded infarct-related artery.[44] However, these results can only apply to patients with an occluded infarct-related artery 3 to 28 days after an acute myocardial infarction and PCI was not guided by ischemia nor myocardial viability testing.[45]

Baks and colleagues[46] studied 27 patients who underwent successful CTO recanalization with DES and whom had CMR before and after intervention. They found that segmental wall thickening (SWT) improved most significantly in segments with less than 25% transmural extent of infarction by LGE CMR. A recent single-center prospective study used stress CMR to guide CTO intervention on candidate patients with stable angina and estimated occlusion duration of greater than or equal to 3 months believed to be suitable for recanalization based on review of their coronary angiogram.[45] Those believed to have viability based on a criteria of less than 75% transmural LGE in most of the CTO segments and an inducible perfusion defect, proceeded with intervention and underwent repeat CMR 3 months after successful CTO recanalization. Myocardial perfusion reserve improved significantly in the CTO region (2.3 ± 0.9 vs 1.8 ± 0.72; $P = .02$) with complete or near-complete resolution of CTO-related perfusion defect in 90% of patients, LV EF increased from $63 \pm 13\%$ to $67 \pm 17\%$ ($P<.0001$), end-systolic volume decreased from 65 ± 38 to 56 ± 38 mL ($P<.001$), and the patients showed improvement in symptoms based on the Seattle Angina Questionnaire score 3 months after CTO PCI.

Kirschbaum and colleagues[47] evaluated LV function recovery with CMR preprocedure, 5 months, and 3 years after CTO percutaneous recanalization. SWT significantly improved at 5-month follow-up ($P<.001$) in those with less than 25% transmural infarct but not in those with 25% to 75% transmural infarct ($P = .89$). However, at 3 years there was an improvement in SWT in those with 25% to 75% transmural infarct suggesting that the recovery time of dysfunction myocardium was related to the extent of damage on a cellular level.

SUMMARY

Patients with obstructive CAD and severe LV dysfunction are known to have a poor prognosis. Those who can undergo successful revascularization have a decrease in mortality. The goal of viability testing is to identify whether there is significant viable myocardium that would likely result in an improved outcome with coronary revascularization. If no significant

viability is identified, the risk for perioperative morbidity is likely higher than the gain from revascularization. Table 1 summarizes the advantages and disadvantages of the most common modalities currently available for assessment of viability. It is imperative that interventional cardiologists understand the advantages and limitations of each method when trying to make decisions on revascularization. Viability testing is not needed in all patients with ischemic cardiomyopathy, such as those with angina or documented ischemia, which by definition is associated with viable myocardium. However, more studies have recently been published in viability assessment before CTO interventions, a growing field with some controversy as how to manage these lesions. There remains room for clinical trials using viability testing to guide patient management.

REFERENCES

1. Burns RJ, Gibbons RJ, Yi Q, et al. The relationships of left ventricular ejection fraction, end-systolic volume index and infarct size to six-month mortality after hospital discharge following myocardial infarction treated by thrombolysis. J Am Coll Cardiol 2002;39:30–6.
2. Møller JE, Egstrup K, Køber L, et al. Prognostic importance of systolic and diastolic function after acute myocardial infarction. Am Heart J 2003;145:147–53.
3. Marwick TH. The viable myocardium: epidemiology, detection, and clinical implications. Lancet 1998;351:815–9.
4. Helfant RH, Pine R, Meister SG, et al. Nitroglycerin to unmask reversible asynergy. Correlation with post coronary bypass ventriculography. Circulation 1974;50:108–13.
5. Dyke SH, Cohn PF, Gorlin R, et al. Detection of residual myocardial function in coronary artery disease using post-extra systolic potentiation. Circulation 1974;50:694–9.
6. Bonow RO, Maurer G, Lee KL, et al. Myocardial viability and survival in ischemic left ventricular dysfunction. N Engl J Med 2011;364:1617–25.
7. Camici PG, Prasad SK, Rimoldi OE. Stunning, hibernation, and assessment of myocardial viability. Circulation 2008;117:103–14.
8. Braunwald E, Kloner RA. The stunned myocardium: prolonged, postischemic ventricular dysfunction. Circulation 1982;66:1146–9.
9. Di Carli MF, Asgarzadie F, Schelbert HR, et al. Quantitative relation between myocardial viability and improvement in heart failure symptoms after revascularization in patients with ischemic cardiomyopathy. Circulation 1995;92:3436–44.

10. Eitzman D, Al-Aouar Z, Kanter HL, et al. Clinical outcome of patients with advanced coronary artery disease after viability studies with positron emission tomography. J Am Coll Cardiol 1992;20: 559–65.

11. Bhat A, Gan GC, Tan TC, et al. Myocardial viability: from proof of concept to clinical practice. Cardiol Res Pract 2016;2016:1020818.

12. Bax JJ, Schinkel AF, Boersma E, et al. Extensive left ventricular remodeling does not allow viable myocardium to improve in left ventricular ejection fraction after revascularization and is associated with worse long-term prognosis. Circulation 2004; 110:II18–22.

13. Velazquez EJ, Lee KL, Jones RH, et al. Coronary-artery bypass surgery in patients with ischemic cardiomyopathy. N Engl J Med 2016;374:1511–20.

14. Desideri A, Cortigiani L, Christen AI, et al. The extent of perfusion-F18-fluorodeoxyglucose positron emission tomography mismatch determines mortality in medically treated patients with chronic ischemic left ventricular dysfunction. J Am Coll Cardiol 2005;46:1264–9.

15. Schinkel AF, Bax JJ, Poldermans D, et al. Hibernating myocardium: diagnosis and patient outcomes. Curr Probl Cardiol 2007;32:375–410.

16. Allman KC, Shaw LJ, Hachamovitch R, et al. Myocardial viability testing and impact of revascularization on prognosis in patients with coronary artery disease and left ventricular dysfunction: a meta-analysis. J Am Coll Cardiol 2002;39:1151–8.

17. Udelson JE, Coleman PS, Metherall J, et al. Predicting recovery of severe regional ventricular dysfunction. Comparison of resting scintigraphy with 201Tl and 99mTc-sestamibi. Circulation 1994;89:2552–61.

18. Henzlova MJ, Duvall WL, Einstein AJ, et al. ASNC imaging guidelines for SPECT nuclear cardiology procedures: stress, protocols, and tracers. J Nucl Cardiol 2016;23:606–39.

19. Kitsiou AN, Srinivasan G, Quyyumi AA, et al. Stress-induced reversible and mild-to-moderate irreversible thallium defects: are they equally accurate for predicting recovery of regional left ventricular function after revascularization? Circulation 1998;98: 501–8.

20. Buckley O, Di Carli M. Predicting benefit from revascularization in patients with ischemic heart failure: imaging of myocardial ischemia and viability. Circulation 2011;123:444–50.

21. Pellikka PA, Nagueh SF, Elhendy AA, et al, American Society of Echocardiography. American Society of Echocardiography recommendations for performance, interpretation, and application of stress echocardiography. J Am Soc Echocardiogr 2007;20:1021–41.

22. Cwajg JM, Cwajg E, Nagueh SF, et al. End-diastolic wall thickness as a predictor of recovery of function in myocardial hibernation: relation to rest-redistribution T1-201 tomography and dobutamine stress echocardiography. J Am Coll Cardiol 2000; 35:1152–61.

23. Biagini E, Galema TW, Schinkel AF, et al. Myocardial wall thickness predicts recovery of contractile function after primary coronary intervention for acute myocardial infarction. J Am Coll Cardiol 2004;43:1489–93.

24. Bax JJ, Poldermans D, Elhendy A, et al. Sensitivity, specificity, and predictive accuracies of various noninvasive techniques for detecting hibernating myocardium. Curr Probl Cardiol 2001;26:147–81.

25. Nagueh SF, Mikati I, Weilbaecher D, et al. Relation of the contractile reserve of hibernating myocardium to myocardial structure in humans. Circulation 1999;100:490–6.

26. Afridi I, Grayburn PA, Panza JA, et al. Myocardial viability during dobutamine echocardiography predicts survival in patients with coronary artery disease and severe left ventricular systolic dysfunction. J Am Coll Cardiol 1998;32:921–6.

27. Meluzin J, Cerny J, Frelich M, et al. Prognostic value of the amount of dysfunctional but viable myocardium in revascularized patients with coronary artery disease and left ventricular dysfunction. investigators of this multicenter study. J Am Coll Cardiol 1998;32:912–20.

28. Afridi I, Kleiman NS, Raizner AE, et al. Dobutamine echocardiography in myocardial hibernation. optimal dose and accuracy in predicting recovery of ventricular function after coronary angioplasty. Circulation 1995;91:663–70.

29. Cornel JH, Bax JJ, Elhendy A, et al. Biphasic response to dobutamine predicts improvement of global left ventricular function after surgical revascularization in patients with stable coronary artery disease: Implications of time course of recovery on diagnostic accuracy. J Am Coll Cardiol 1998; 31:1002–10.

30. Perrone-Filardi P, Pace L, Prastaro M, et al. Dobutamine echocardiography predicts improvement of hypoperfused dysfunctional myocardium after revascularization in patients with coronary artery disease. Circulation 1995;91:2556–65.

31. Collidge TA, Thomson PC, Mark PB, et al. Gadolinium-enhanced MR imaging and nephrogenic systemic fibrosis: retrospective study of a renal replacement therapy cohort. Radiology 2007;245: 168–75.

32. Wang Y, Alkasab TK, Narin O, et al. Incidence of nephrogenic systemic fibrosis after adoption of restrictive gadolinium-based contrast agent guidelines. Radiology 2011;260:105–11.

33. Indik JH, Gimbel JR, Abe H, et al. 2017 HRS expert consensus statement on magnetic resonance imaging and radiation exposure in patients with

cardiovascular implantable electronic devices. Heart Rhythm 2017;14:e97–153.

34. Kim RJ, Wu E, Rafael A, et al. The use of contrast-enhanced magnetic resonance imaging to identify reversible myocardial dysfunction. N Engl J Med 2000;343:1445–53.

35. Klein C, Nekolla SG, Bengel FM, et al. Assessment of myocardial viability with contrast-enhanced magnetic resonance imaging: comparison with positron emission tomography. Circulation 2002; 105:162–7.

36. Romero J, Xue X, Gonzalez W, et al. CMR imaging assessing viability in patients with chronic ventricular dysfunction due to coronary artery disease: a meta-analysis of prospective trials. JACC Cardiovasc Imaging 2012;5:494–508.

37. Shah DJ, Kim HW, James O, et al. Prevalence of regional myocardial thinning and relationship with myocardial scarring in patients with coronary artery disease. JAMA 2013;309:909–18.

38. Dilsizian V, Bacharach SL, Beanlands RS, et al. ASNC imaging guidelines/SNMMI procedure standard for positron emission tomography (PET) nuclear cardiology procedures. J Nucl Cardiol 2016; 23:1187–226.

39. Schelbert HR, Beanlands R, Bengel F, et al. PET myocardial perfusion and glucose metabolism imaging: part 2-guidelines for interpretation and reporting. J Nucl Cardiol 2003;10:557–71.

40. Tillisch J, Brunken R, Marshall R, et al. Reversibility of cardiac wall-motion abnormalities predicted by positron tomography. N Engl J Med 1986;314: 884–8.

41. Beanlands RSB, Nichol G, Huszti E, et al. F-18-fluorodeoxyglucose positron emission tomography imaging-assisted management of patients with severe left ventricular dysfunction and suspected coronary disease: a randomized, controlled trial (PARR-2). J Am Coll Cardiol 2007;50:2002–12.

42. Panza JA, Bonow RO. Ischemia and viability testing in ischemic heart disease: the available evidence and how we interpret it. JACC Cardiovasc Imaging 2017;10:365–7.

43. Chareonthaitawee P, Gersh BJ, Panza JA. Is viability imaging still relevant in 2012? JACC Cardiovasc Imaging 2012;5:550–8.

44. Hochman JS, Lamas GA, Buller CE, et al. Coronary intervention for persistent occlusion after myocardial infarction. N Engl J Med 2006;355: 2395–407.

45. Bucciarelli-Ducci C, Auger D, Di Mario C, et al. CMR guidance for recanalization of coronary chronic total occlusion. JACC Cardiovasc Imaging 2016;9:547–56.

46. Baks T, van Geuns R, Duncker DJ, et al. Prediction of left ventricular function after drug-eluting stent implantation for chronic total coronary occlusions. J Am Coll Cardiol 2006;47:721–5.

47. Kirschbaum SW, Baks T, van den Ent M, et al. Evaluation of left ventricular function three years after percutaneous recanalization of chronic total coronary occlusions. Am J Cardiol 2008;101:179–85.

Computed Tomography for Left Atrial Appendage Occlusion Case Planning

Marvin H. Eng, MD*, Dee Dee Wang, MD

KEYWORDS

• Atrial fibrillation • Left atrial appendage • Thromboprophylaxis • Computed tomography

KEY POINTS

- Because of its variable structure and anatomic location, accurate analysis of the left atrial appendage (LAA) relies on multiple imaging planes; therefore a complete characterization of the LAA by TEE imaging can be challenging and highly operator dependent.
- Computed tomography (CT) is sensitive for LAA thrombus, with high negative predictive value; however, given its relatively low specificity, TEE is required for confirmation.
- Compared with CT, TEE systematically underestimates LAA ostial dimension and LAA depth; CT also identifies patients in whom Watchman LAA closure is feasible but are excluded by TEE, most commonly because of LAA depth that is sufficient but undetected by echocardiography.
- Preprocedural CT evaluation appears to improve procedural efficiency (ie, sheath selection and device size) compared with TEE guidance alone; this could improve procedural complication rates.
- Other potential benefits of preprocedural CT imaging of the LAA include identifying the coplanar viewing angle on left atrial angiography and 3-dimensional printing for ex-vivo device implant simulation.

INTRODUCTION

The left atrial appendage (LAA) has been under intense scrutiny since being identified as a source for systemic thromboembolism, most notably stroke. Approximately 795,000 patients in the United States experience a new or recurrent stroke and 87% of strokes are ischemic.[1] Atrial arrhythmias, especially atrial fibrillation remain a major contributor of ischemic stroke, as 23.5% of ischemic strokes in patients from the ages of 80 to 89 years are attributed to atrial fibrillation.[2,3] Review of several echocardiographic and surgical observations have confirmed that approximately 91% of thrombi in cases of nonvalvular atrial fibrillation originates from the atrial appendage; therefore, efforts have been directed toward obliterating this space in hopes of mitigating strokes.[4] Although anticoagulation can prevent stroke, for various reasons many patients are not treated, and several investigative trials have focused on mechanically obliterating the LAA.[5–7] Percutaneous occlusion of the atrial appendage has been a focus of research recently and with the maturation of endovascular devices, detailed anatomic analysis of the left atrial appendage has come to the forefront of cardiology in the interest of optimizing the safety and efficacy of appendage interventions. Both 3-dimensional

Dr M.H. Eng is a proctor for Edwards Lifesciences. Dr D.D. Wang is a coinventor on a patent application assigned to Henry Ford Health System, on software for LAA planning.
Division of Cardiology, Center for Structural Heart Disease, Henry Ford Hospital, Detroit, MI 48236, USA
* Corresponding author. 2799 West Grand Boulevard, Clara Ford Pavilion, Room 434, Detroit, MI 48202.
E-mail address: meng1@hfhs.org

Intervent Cardiol Clin 7 (2018) 367–378
https://doi.org/10.1016/j.iccl.2018.03.003

echocardiography and contrast computed to-mography (CT) are the primary modalities considered. This article focuses on the use and impact of the latter.

The LAA is a complex, multiform structure with great variability across individuals. LAA may have single, double or several small lobes, and LAA size does not correlate to body habitus or gender. Most appendages (54%) have 2 lobes; approximately 25 percent have 3 lobes, and 20% have 1 lobe.[8] Above 20 years of age, body size, age and gender do not correlate to atrial appendage size; however, there is a weak relationship with height.[8] One can broadly categorize the various morphologic shapes into windsock, chicken-wing, cactus, and cauliflower based on CT characterization; however, the authors find this categorization an oversimplification of the morphologic variability found in appendage anatomy (Fig. 1).[9] Retrospective review of a large cohort of patients with left atrial CT scans revealed that morphology may play a role in thromboembolic risk. Chicken-wing appendages were found to have the lowest incidence of thromboemboli, while the rate of stroke in cauliflower appendages were increased by eight-fold.[10] Morphologic variability extends to appendage ostia, as some are oval-shaped, while others are triangular, teardrop, foot-like, and round-shaped.[8,9] Given the thin-walled, compliant nature of this anatomic structure, a detailed understanding of relevant dimensions is necessary for safe implantation of devices.

Initial interventional treatment was fraught with complications. The WATCHMAN (Boston Scientific, Natick, Massachusetts), was the first device in the United States to undergo prospective clinical investigations and has the most complete dataset

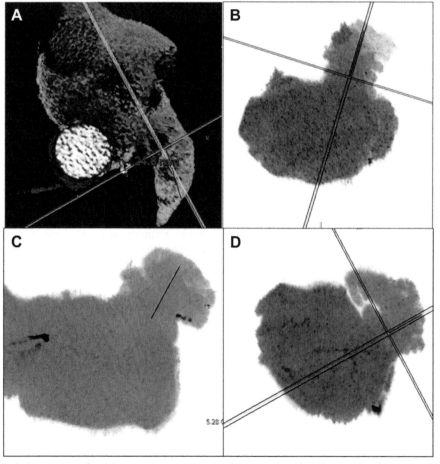

Fig. 1. Morphologic types of atrial appendages as previously categorized by Wang and colleagues. (A) Windsock shaped appendage. (B) Cactus shaped appendage. (C) Cauliflower shaped appendage. (D) Chicken-wing shaped appendage.

to analyze. These studies showed significant rates of periprocedural pericardial effusions and tamponade; analysis of the PROTECT-AF (WATCHMAN Left Atrial Appendage System for Embolic Protection in Patients with Atrial Fibrillation) trial showed an 8.7% rate of 7-day procedural complications that decreased to 4.8% in PREVAIL (Prospective Randomized Evaluation of the Watchman Left Atrial Appendage Closure Device In Patients with Atrial Fibrillation vs Long Term Warfarin Therapy). Although some of these events may be from an early operator learning curve, some of this safety signal may be related to incomplete knowledge and understanding of appendage anatomy.[11,12] Moreover, operators in PREVAIL used 1.8 devices per case, suggesting that improvements could be made in device or catheter selection to decrease the number of exchanges inside the left atrium, thus minimizing opportunities for error and complications.

Although characterization and imaging of the LAA is traditionally performed with transesophageal echocardiography, computed tomography (CT) enables a more detailed characterization of this structure. Analyzing the LAA for the purposes of device deployment requires careful inspection of the distance of the ostium to the distal tip of the major left atrial appendage lobe, size of the ostium, and an understanding of the morphology. Because of the highly variable structure with the propensity to be multilobar, accurate analysis of the appendage relies on multiple imaging planes, and the completeness of TEE imaging can be highly operator dependent.[8] CT prior to the arrival of catheterization laboratory enables implanters with the foreknowledge of presence of thrombus, atrial-caval anatomy, appendage morphology, and deployment angles. Three-dimensional printing of the left atrium can be used for simulation of ex-vivo implantation (Table 1). One advantage of CT is that the patient does not need to be fasting, thereby preventing dehydration, as volume depletion leads to underestimation of appendage dimensions.[13]

TECHNIQUE FOR LEFT ATRIAL APPENDAGE COMPUTED TOMOGRAPHY ANALYSIS

The CT scanning protocol, generation of the 3-dimensional rendering, and data extraction have been previously described and bear similarities to CT acquisitions for the aortic and mitral valve.[14] Briefly, preprocedure imaging utilizes a contrast-enhanced, retrospectively electrocardiogram-gated CTA acquisition without electrocardiogram (ECG) dose

modulation using at minimum a 64-slice scanner. Heart rate is controlled for a goal of less than 90 bpm to optimize scanning, and the patient must be able to cooperate with a breath hold. Iodinated contrast is injected at a rate of 4 mL/s, for a total volume of 80 mL via an 18-gauge peripheral intravenous line. After image acquisition, CT DICOM (digital imaging and communications in medicine) data are analyzed using a software package capable of multiplanar reconstruction. Our center utilizes Vitrea (Vital Images, Minnetonka, Minnesota) and Mimics (Materialise Leuven, Belgium) (see Table 1). Raw CT DICOM data containing the previously mentioned diastolic phase of the LAA are exported to specialized computer-aided-design (CAD) segmentation software (Mimics; Materialise, Leuven, Belgium), where the blood volume of the left atrium, LAA, aortic annulus, and rims of the SVC and IVC are manually segmented and 3-dimensionally printed (see Table 1). The segmentation technique (see Table 1) shown here has been previously reported and optimized for the WATCHMAN device, but other published literature show that CT planning has been used for alternate appendage occluders including the Amplatz Cardiac Plug (Abbott Vascular, Abbott Park, Illinois) or Amulet device (Abbott Vascular, Abbott Park, Illinois).[14]

APPENDAGE ANALYSIS AND LANDING ZONE IDENTIFICATION FOR WATCHMAN IMPLANTATION
Identifying True Systole Computed Tomography
Utilizing a 5% to 95% reconstructed valve cine series of the CT, the LAA is analyzed in 10% reconstructed R-R intervals in a CT-rendered 4-dimensioal cine clip. The selection of the mid-late systolic phase for the LAA should be performed by a physician experienced in 3-dimensional analysis and multiplanar segmentation and reconstruction.

Identifying the Landing Zone: How to Select the WATCHMAN Device
Key to device selection for the LAA is identifying the zone of the LAA that will seat the WATCHMAN device with optimal device stability and coaxial positioning to the main body of the appendage (Fig. 2). Sizing of the LAA typically occurs at the junction between the left atrium (LA) and LAA interface, and most measurements use the plane contiguous with the superior and inferior border of the appendage ostium (see Fig. 2A). However, WATCHMAN devices typically align themselves to the long-axis centerline of the

Table 1
Left atrial appendage segmentation protocol

Sizing the LAA landing zone	Load the 0%–95% valve series of the LAA into CT viewer. Identify the phase that corresponds to mid- to end-left ventricular systolic filling that corresponds best to maximal end-LAA diastolic filling. In the coronal cross-sections, place the cross hairs on the LAA.	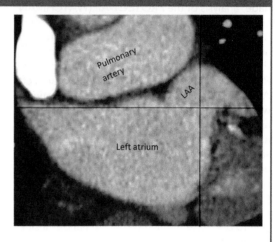
	In a curved multiplanar reformat plane, within the coronal window, double oblique the sagittal cross hairs (blue) to the direction of the main lobe of the LAA.	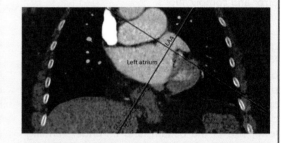
	In the sagittal window, within a curved multiplanar reformat plane, advance the cross hairs to the level of the proximal left circumflex (LCx) artery takeoff from the left anterior descending artery. Then, double oblique the coronal cross hairs (green) to the direction of the main lobe of the LAA (commonly runs parallel to the course of the left anterior descending (LAD) artery).	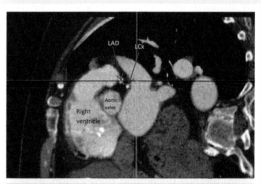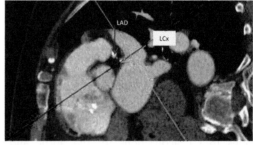

(continued on next page)

On the axial cross-sections, measure the maximal and minimal diameters, area, and circumference of the LAA landing zone.

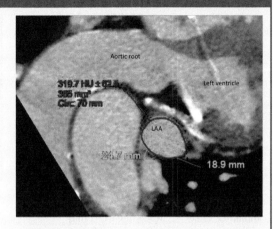

Identifying the maximal length of the LAA landing zone to distal tip of the main lobe of the LAA

Identify the maximal length or depth of the LAA from the landing zone to the distal LAA tip of in the sagittal and coronal views, and record the largest value. (Scroll in and out of the identified view to ensure maximal length is accounted for.)

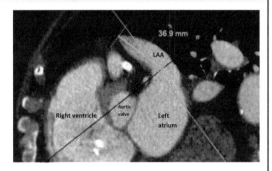

Generating the length of the WATCHMAN delivery sheath

Adjust the length measurement to equal the maximal width of the WATCHMAN device selected (per the sizing guidelines from the WATCHMAN DFU). In this patient, a 24.7 mm maximal width diameter corresponds to selection of a 27 mm WATCHMAN device, and hence delivery sheath depth of approximately 27 mm (plus or minus 0.5 mm to account for distal delivery tip plastic tricut length and presence or absence of LAA pedunculations protruding into site of catheter positioning).

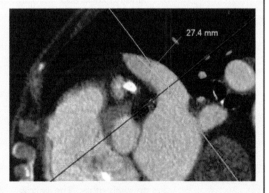

(continued on next page)

C-arm Angles	Segment the LAA, LA, into a transparent 3-dimensional volume image. In the 3-dimensional window, align the axial (red) and sagittal (blue) planes to intersect perpendicular to each other. Show the delivery sheath length in the 3-dimensional image (pink line).	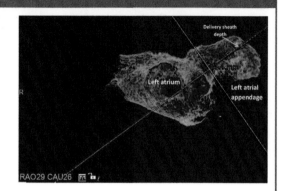
Implanter Case Plan	Apply inverted mip (maximal intensity projection) to the 3-dimensional volume to project the 3-dimensional image in a black-white radiograph simulation. Load the image screenshot into Microsoft Powerpoint, apply 'insert art tool' and overlay the cross hairs with a bracket and line (over the demarcated delivery sheath) to simulate the WATCHMAN device landing zone and delivery sheath depth positioning.	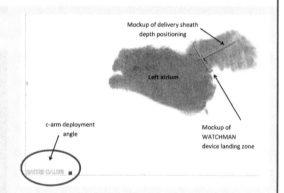
Interventional Imaging Case Plan (TEE 45° view)	Segment the aortic annulus, proximal left anterior descending and circumflex artery into the 3-dimensional volume. Adjust the image to bring the aortic valve centered and anterior. Adjust the axial (red) and coronal (green) cross hairs to intersect perpendicular to each other. The yellow arrow depicts delivery sheath positioning when imaging in the 2-dimensional TEE mid-esophageal short-axis view of the aortic valve.	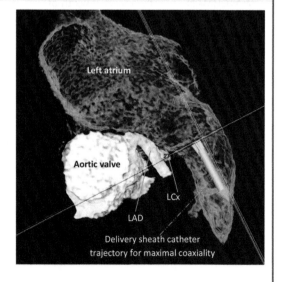

(continued on next page)

TEE 135° View	Rotate the 3-dimensional image along the sagittal plane (red cross-hair) until the aorta is at 3 PM and anterior to the LAA. Remove the aortic root from the 3-dimensional volume. With the LAA pointing toward 6 PM, the yellow arrow depicts the delivery catheter and sheath tip position for maximal catheter coaxial position to optimize WATCHMAN implantation. The sagittal plane (red cross hair) now depicts the landing zone to be shown by 2-dimensional TEE in the 135° view.	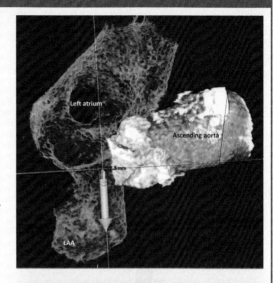
		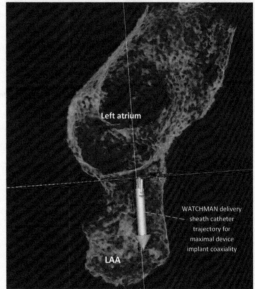
3-Dimensional Print Assisted Type Of Delivery Catheter (single, anterior, double curve) selection	3-dimensional prints of patient's specific LA, LAA anatomy were generated to assist in bench-test selection of catheter curvature for device implantation.	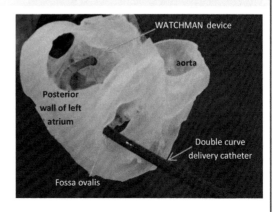

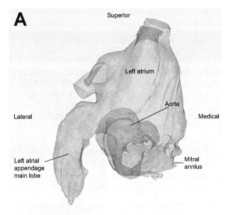

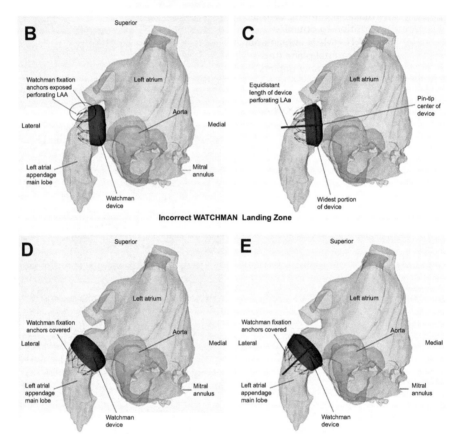

Fig. 2. Defining the LAA landing zone. The mid-to-end left ventricular systolic phase corresponding to maximal LAA diastolic filling is identified and segmented into a CAD 3-dimensional volume image of the patient's specific anatomy (A). Traditional sizing of the LAA typically occurs at the junction between the LA and LAA interface. However, WATCHMAN devices typically align themselves to the long-axis centerline of the appendage, and the device shoulders do not necessarily match the same plane as the LA and LAA interface (B). Virtually implanting that sized device in the same plane as the assumed LA-LAA interface results in a simulated canted deployment that does not conform to the borders of the appendage and misrepresents the final alignment of the device (C). Therefore, measurements at the LA-LAA interface could differ significantly from a more accurately simulated landing zone depending on the trajectory of the device deployment. Once the main lobe of the LAA is identified and the WATCHMAN device is primarily aligned to the long axis of the lobe and not the plane of the ostium, the measurement the plane near the ostium orthogonal to the long axis better reflects the implantation zone dimensions. The "T" verifies that there is equal width and depth to ensure: (1) all WATCHMAN fixation anchors come in contact with the inner surface of the LAA; (2) there is sufficient seal around the device cap; and (3) major outpouchings or pedunculations are covered distal to the device landing zone (D, E).

appendage, and the device shoulders do not necessarily match the same plane as the LA and LAA interface (see Fig. 2B). Virtually implanting that sized device in the same plane as the assumed LA-LAA interface results in a simulated canted deployment that does not conform to the borders of the appendage and may misrepresent the final alignment of the device (see Fig. 2C). Therefore, measurements at the LA-LAA interface could differ significantly from a more accurately simulated landing zone depending on the trajectory of the device deployment. Once the main lobe of the LAA is identified and the simulated WATCHMAN device is primarily aligned to the long axis of the lobe and not the plane of the ostium, the measurement of the plane near the ostium orthogonal to the long axis is described as the true ostium (see Fig. 2D, E). On CT, in the coronal and sagittal cross-sections, the cross hairs are aligned in each respective plane perpendicular to the blood flow of the main lobe of the true ostium of the LAA. Once the true ostium of the LAA landing zone is identified, the maximal/minimal diameters, area, and perimeter of the LAA are obtained in the multiplanar reformatted double oblique axial projection (see Table 1). Maximal length of the LAA is defined as a point from the center of the true ostium of the LAA to the most distal contiguous portion of the LAA in the form of a straight line circumscribed within the blood volume of the LAA.

Creating the 3-Dimensional Print

Raw CT DICOM data containing the previously mentioned systolic phase of the LAA are exported to specialized CAD segmentation software (Mimics; Materialise, Leuven, Belgium). The blood volume of the LA, LAA, aortic annulus, and rims of the SVC and IVC are manually segmented and 3-dimensionally printed. When there is difficulty in conceptualizing and identifying the true ostium of the LAA on CT imaging, a physical WATCHMAN device is implanted *ex vivo* in the patient's 3-dimensionally printed LAA to simulate device positioning (see Table 1).

COMPUTED TOMOGRAPHY OF THE LEFT ATRIAL APPENDAGE FOR THROMBUS DETECTION

Validation of CT for identifying atrial thrombus has been previously performed and enables CT to circumvent transesophageal echocardiogram assessment for not only device sizing, but clot as well. Retrospective review of CT and TEE done within 7 days of each other showed a sensitivity of 93%, specificity 85%, positive predictive

value (PPV) of 31%, and negative predictive value (NPV) of 99%.[15] Another study with 402 patients recapitulated these results with comparable values (sensitivity 100%, specificity 92%, NPV 100% and PPV 23%).[16] Therefore, we can conclude that CT offers excellent sensitivity with good negative predictive value but the current specificity requires TEE to confirm the presence of thrombus.

COMPUTED TOMOGRAPHY VERSUS TEE FOR LEFT ATRIAL APPENDAGE DIMENSIONS

Comparative studies reproducibly show that CT measurements of the appendage diameter and length typically exceed that of 2-dimensional TEE and fluoroscopy. There was inconsistent correlation for CT compared with TEE (r = 0.49–0.8) for the LAA ostium; however, the correlation for appendage length was poor (r = 0.56 CTA/TEE).[17,18] When comparing with fluoroscopy, CT again still had the largest measurements, with a correlation R-value of 0.71 to 0.81 for width, but again the greatest difference was observed in the length (R = 0.28).[18] The authors surmise that the curvilinear nature of the appendage lobe length is difficult to appreciate with TEE, and sampling errors are easy to make depending on the shape of the major lobe. Although the absolute differences between CT and TEE measurements for ostium were moderate; 1 to 3 mm differences in appendage width can impact sizing, especially in WATCHMAN implantations given the small ranges for the manufacturer's sizing guide.[19]

Similarly, in the Henry Ford pilot study of using CT for LAA occlusion case planning, the authors' observations concurred that TEE routinely underestimates LAA dimensions.[14] This retrospective series showed that compared with CT, TEE undersizes the LAA maximal width and length by 2.7 plus or minus 2.2 mm and 4.0 plus or minus 5.8 mm, respectively. Even when comparing 3-dimensional echocardiographic datasets to CT, the CT still measures larger by 2.3 plus or minus 3.0 mm.[14] The ramifications of undersizing are significant: by using 2-dimensional TEE maximal width, 62.3% (33/53) of the patients would have received the incorrect initial device and require upsizing to a larger device size intraprocedurally. If not for CT, 12 of 53 patients would have been inappropriately excluded from WATCHMAN implantation either due to width (3 of 53) or length (9 of 53) underestimation.[14] As a result of more accurate LAA measurements, only 1 size of occluder was used for all of the cases. Because of operator challenges to deployment depth and need for recapturing WATCHMAN devices, the average number of devices utilized in this cohort was 1.245 devices with a 100% implantation success. No major complications such as pericardial effusions, perforations, or device embolizations occurred in this 53-patient series. All device exchanges in the LA pose a threat to increasing procedural complications; CT guidance, by minimizing device and catheter exchanges, can hopefully further improve procedural outcomes.

ADDITIONAL PROCEDURAL ADVANTAGES WITH COMPUTED TOMOGRAPHY GUIDANCE

Additional information that CT provides includes coplanar viewing angle (Fig. 3). Unlike calcified aortic valves and transcatheter aortic valve replacement, there are no radiographic markers to help delineate the coplanar view during the procedure.[20] Usually when performing angiography, imaging angles are changed to minimize foreshortening and overlap of other angiographically overlapped structures, most notably in coronary angiography. However, the LAA is entirely a soft tissue structure, and the angiographic projections that minimize foreshortening of the appendage length often do no match the coplanar angle for the ostium of the appendage.[14] In a procedure where minimizing the number of exchanges and catheter exchanges helps avoid complications, simplifying the procedure to 1 catheter, 1 device, and 1 deployment should enhance safety. Furthermore, narrowing the number of angiographic projections minimizes contrast and radiation exposure, another quality marker and safety measure in the catheterization laboratory.

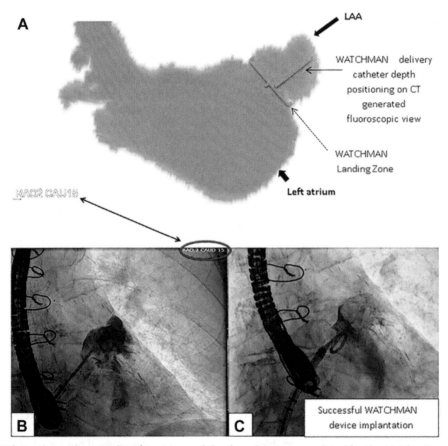

Fig. 3. Defining the coplanar angle. After sizing and depth analysis are completed for the LAA landing zone, the LAA, LA, and any pertinent adjacent anatomic landmark structure (eg, transcatheter valves, sternotomy wires) are segmented and projected into inverted maximal-intensity projection to simulate the intraprocedural LAA angiogram (A). Appropriate C-arm angles are generated and demonstrated on the actual day of a successful procedural implantation with baseline LAA angiography at those angles (B), and final device implantation corresponds to the proposed case plan provided by CT (C).

Another advantage of CT data includes creation of physical models that can be used for *ex-vivo* bench testing of device fit and catheter suitability (see Table 1). The 3-dimensional data from a CT scan can be exported to CAD software, but the data must be manually manipulated and then sent to a 3-dimensional printer for creation of an actual physical model. Using this heart replica, catheters and devices can be fit-tested and tried prior to starting a procedure. Therefore, many assumptions about coaxial catheter and accurate device selection can be investigated without manipulation in the body, instead of a dogmatic progression from the same standard guiding catheter and changing catheters after failed attempts.

POSTPROCEDURAL DEVICE SURVEILLANCE

Postimplant surveillance is an additional utility of CT. It appears to be more sensitive than TEE for detection of postimplant peridevice leaks, as it detected leaks in 62% of patients post-Amplatzer cardiac plug implantation, while TEE only detected leaks in 36% of patients.[21] All of the leaks were small (mean 1.5 plus or minus 1.4 mm) and localized to the postero-superior and postero-inferior portion of the appendage. This rate of leak detection is consistent with that detected in a single-center, 45-patient mixed-cohort post-ACP and WATCHMAN implantations with a 62% rate.[22] In addition to peridevice leaks, device thrombus and embolization were detected as well. Although the gold standard for device leaks remains TEE, CT may become an acceptable substitute so long as the significance of the leak is kept in context: postprocedure leaks less than 5 mm that were detected by TEE, a less sensitive test than CT, were not associated with subsequent thromboembolic events in the PROTECT-AF randomized clinical trial.[23]

LIMITATIONS OF COMPUTED TOMOGRAPHY GUIDANCE

Although there are many advantages to using CT data, its use may not be broadly applicable. For instance, a CT-angiogram requires an additional dose of radiation and contrast, which may be harmful or undesirable in some patients. Furthermore, processing the data is laborious, and not all centers may have the resources or infrastructure to manually analyze additional CT data. Creating 3-dimensional models is yet an additional infrastructure and financial challenge that may not be easily met in today's health care environment. Repeating a gated CT-angiogram for the purposes of device surveillance again provides an additive dose of radiation, and contrast and should be carefully considered. Nevertheless, improving how to use advanced imaging data represents yet another iterative step of progress in the field of interventional cardiology.

SUMMARY

TEE will remain the cornerstone of performing complex structural heart procedures, but the role of CT in treating aortic valve disease, mitral valve disease, and now LAA occlusion is becoming indispensable.[14,24,25] The breadth and complexity of structural heart disease interventions continue to expand, and improving the safety, quality, and success of percutaneous interventions will depend heavily on advanced imaging. Increasing complexity of structural heart interventions calls for thorough preparation and flawless execution.

REFERENCES

1. Benjamin EJ, Blaha MJ, Chiuve SE, et al. Heart disease and stroke statistics—2017 update: a report from the American Heart Association. Circulation 2017;135(10):e146–603.
2. Wolf PA, Abbott RD, Kannel WB. Atrial fibrillation as an independent risk factor for stroke: the Framingham Study. Stroke 1991;22(8):983–8.
3. Wang TJ, Massaro JM, Levy D, et al. A risk score for predicting stroke or death in individuals with new-onset atrial fibrillation in the community: the Framingham Heart Study. JAMA 2003;290(8):1049–56.
4. Blackshear JL, Odell JA. Appendage obliteration to reduce stroke in cardiac surgical patients with atrial fibrillation. Ann Thorac Surg 1996;61(2):755–9.
5. Go AS, Mozaffarian D, Roger VL, et al. Heart disease and stroke statistics—2014 update. a report from the American Heart Association. Circulation 2014;129(3):e28–292.
6. Reddy VY, Sievert H, Halperin J, et al. Percutaneous left atrial appendage closure vs warfarin for atrial fibrillation: a randomized clinical trial. JAMA 2014; 312(19):1988–98.
7. Reddy VY, Doshi SK, Kar S, et al. 5-year outcomes after left atrial appendage closure: from the PREVAIL and PROTECT AF trials. J Am Coll Cardiol 2017;70(24):2964–75.
8. Veinot JP, Harrity PJ, Gentile F, et al. Anatomy of the normal left atrial appendage. a quantitative study of age-related changes in 500 autopsy

hearts: implications for echocardiographic examination. Circulation 1997;96(9):3112–5.

9. Wang Y, Di Biase L, Horton RP, et al. Left atrial appendage studied by computed tomography to help planning for appendage closure device placement. J Cardiovasc Electrophysiol 2010; 21(9):973–82.

10. Di Biase L, Santangeli P, Anselmino M, et al. Does the left atrial appendage morphology correlate with the risk of stroke in patients with atrial fibrillation? Results from a multicenter study. J Am Coll Cardiol 2012;60(6):531–8.

11. Reddy VY, Holmes D, Doshi SK, et al. Safety of percutaneous left atrial appendage closure: results from the watchman left atrial appendage system for embolic protection in patients with AF (PROTECT AF) clinical trial and the continued access registry. Circulation 2011;123(4):417–24.

12. Holmes DR Jr, Kar S, Price MJ, et al. Prospective randomized evaluation of the watchman left atrial appendage closure device in patients with atrial fibrillation versus long-term warfarin therapy: the PREVAIL trial. J Am Coll Cardiol 2014;64(1):1–12.

13. Spencer RJ, DeJong P, Fahmy P, et al. Changes in left atrial appendage dimensions following volume loading during percutaneous left atrial appendage closure. JACC Cardiovasc Interv 2015;8(15):1935–41.

14. Wang DD, Eng M, Kupsky D, et al. Application of 3-dimensional computed tomographic image guidance to WATCHMAN implantation and impact on early operator learning curve: single-center experience. JACC Cardiovasc Interv 2016; 9(22):2329–40.

15. Kim YY, Klein AL, Halliburton SS, et al. Left atrial appendage filling defects identified by multidetector computed tomography in patients undergoing radiofrequency pulmonary vein antral isolation: a comparison with transesophageal echocardiography. Am Heart J 2007;154(6):1199–205.

16. Martinez MW, Kirsch J, Williamson EE, et al. Utility of nongated multidetector computed tomography for detection of left atrial thrombus in patients undergoing catheter ablation of atrial fibrillation. JACC Cardiovasc Imaging 2009;2(1):69–76.

17. Budge LP, Shaffer KM, Moorman JR, et al. Analysis of in vivo left atrial appendage morphology in patients with atrial fibrillation: a direct comparison of transesophageal echocardiography, planar cardiac CT, and segmented three-dimensional cardiac CT. J Interv Card Electrophysiol 2008;23(2): 87–93.

18. Saw J, Fahmy P, Spencer R, et al. Comparing measurements of CT angiography, TEE, and fluoroscopy of the left atrial appendage for percutaneous closure. J Cardiovasc Electrophysiol 2016;27(4): 414–22.

19. WATCHMAN left atrial appendage closure device and delivery system [package insert]. Marlborough, MA: Boston Scientific Corporation; 2015.

20. Binder RK, Leipsic J, Wood D, et al. Prediction of optimal deployment projection for transcatheter aortic valve replacement: angiographic 3-dimensional reconstruction of the aortic root versus multidetector computed tomography. Circ Cardiovasc Interv 2012;5(2):247–52.

21. Jaguszewski M, Manes C, Puippe G, et al. Cardiac CT and echocardiographic evaluation of peri-device flow after percutaneous left atrial appendage closure using the AMPLATZER cardiac plug device. Catheter Cardiovasc Interv 2015; 85(2):306–12.

22. Saw J, Fahmy P, DeJong P, et al. Cardiac CT angiography for device surveillance after endovascular left atrial appendage closure. Eur Heart J Cardiovasc Imaging 2015;16(11):1198–206.

23. Viles-Gonzalez JF, Kar S, Douglas P, et al. The clinical impact of incomplete left atrial appendage closure with the watchman device in patients with atrial fibrillation: a PROTECT AF (Percutaneous Closure of the Left Atrial Appendage Versus Warfarin Therapy for Prevention of Stroke in Patients With Atrial Fibrillation) substudy. J Am Coll Cardiol 2012;59(10):923–9.

24. Binder RK, Webb JG, Willson AB, et al. The impact of integration of a multidetector computed tomography annulus area sizing algorithm on outcomes of transcatheter aortic valve replacement: a prospective, multicenter, controlled trial. J Am Coll Cardiol 2013;62(5):431–8.

25. Wang DD, Eng MH, Greenbaum AB, et al. Predicting left ventricular outflow tract obstruction after transcatheter mitral valve replacement (TMVR): initial single center experience. JACC Cardiovasc Imaging 2016. [Epub ahead of print].

Multimodality Imaging of the Tricuspid Valve for Assessment and Guidance of Transcatheter Repair

Dee Dee Wang, MD[a],*, James C. Lee, MD[a],
Brian P. O'Neill, MD[b], William W. O'Neill, MD[a]

KEYWORDS

• Transesophageal echocardiogram • CT • 3D printing • MRI • Tricuspid • Transcatheter

---

KEY POINTS

- The tricuspid valve is a highly complex structure, with variability in the number of leaflets and scallops.
- Transcatheter repair of the tricuspid valve with the MitraClip system is commonly guided by transesophageal echocardiography, but the anterior location of the valve can make identification of regurgitant cause and procedural guidance challenging.
- Retrospectively gated computed tomography (CT) can be used to identify tricuspid leaflet motion, areas of malcoaptation, and commissure-to-commissure gap for the assessment of anatomic suitability for off-label MitraClip implantation.
- CT evaluation is critical for preprocedural planning of transcatheter valve implantation within a degenerated tricuspid bioprosthesis or tricuspid annuloplasty ring.
- Cardiac magnetic resonance imaging may be of value in quantification of right ventricular function and tricuspid regurgitation severity in the absence of echocardiographic datasets.

Transcatheter heart valve (THV) therapies have gained widespread attention in the treatment of aortic and mitral valve disease. Advancements in transcatheter valve technology are now shifting toward tricuspid regurgitation.[1] Multimodality imaging is integral to successful transcatheter tricuspid interventions.

UNDERSTANDING TRICUSPID ANATOMY

The tricuspid valve develops from endocardial cushions and the adjacent myocardium, with delamination of the free leaflets from the myocardium at approximately 8 to 16 weeks of development.[2] In a normal heart, the septal annulus of the tricuspid valve is apically displaced compared with the mitral valve. The

---

Disclosures: Dr D.D. Wang is a consultant for Edwards LifeSciences, Boston Scientific and Materialise. Dr D.D. Wang also provides CT core laboratory services through Henry Ford Hospital to the MITRAL trial, and CT and Echo core laboratory services through Henry Ford Hospital to the NIH-sponsored LAMPOON clinical trial. Dr B. P. O'Neill has received research support from Edwards LifeSciences. Dr W. O'Neill is a consultant for Edwards Life-Sciences. Dr J.C. Lee reports no disclosures.
[a] Center for Structural Heart Disease, Henry Ford Hospital, 2799 West Grand Boulevard, Clara Ford Pavilion 4th Floor, 432, Detroit, MI 48202, USA; [b] Department of Medicine, Section of Cardiology, Temple Heart and Vascular Institute, 3509 North Broad Street, Philadelphia, PA 19140, USA
* Corresponding author.
E-mail address: dwang2@hfhs.org

Intervent Cardiol Clin 7 (2018) 379–386
https://doi.org/10.1016/j.iccl.2018.04.001

tricuspid valve has traditionally been thought to consist of three distinct leaflets: septal, the inferior (or posterior), and the anterior (or anterosuperior). Each of these leaflets is attached via a complex and highly variable network of chordae tendineae and corresponding papillary muscles.[3] Unique to the tricuspid valve, some of the tricuspid chordae insert directly into the right ventricular myocardium.

The name of the tricuspid valve itself may be a misnomer, because it frequently has both fewer and more cusps. Indeed, the frequency of the presence of three cusps has been reported to range from 28% to 62%.[4,5] Some authors have even called into question of whether the tricuspid valve is even tricuspid and demonstrated that the traditional leaflets have numerous variations in scallops within and between leaflets.[6]

PATHOPHYSIOLOGY OF TRICUSPID REGURGITATION

The mechanisms of tricuspid regurgitation can be broadly classified into primary and secondary causes, similar to that of mitral regurgitation. Primary causes are those with a structural valve abnormality. Secondary, or functional, tricuspid regurgitation is related to incomplete leaflet coaptation, frequently driven by right ventricular dilation leading to tricuspid annular dilation. Tricuspid regurgitation leads to a volume load on the right ventricle, which can then drive a feedback loop of progressive ventricular dilation leading to worse tricuspid regurgitation. This means that even primary causes of tricuspid regurgitation will frequently have a secondary/functional component in their later stages. Although the overall prevalence of tricuspid regurgitation is high, its course is not benign. Severity of tricuspid regurgitation has been independently associated with worse survival,[7] and tricuspid regurgitation, left unchecked, can lead to progressive right ventricular dilation and subsequent heart failure.[8]

With the ongoing innovation and development of new transcatheter technologies, historical, simplified characterizations of the tricuspid valve anatomy and function are no longer sufficient. Complementary imaging techniques, such as 3-dimensional (3D) echocardiography, cardiac computed tomography, and cardiovascular magnetic resonance imaging (CMR), are allowing for significant improvements in the noninvasive visualization and characterization of the tricuspid valve. Using the strengths of each technology to accurately diagnose the mechanism and classify the severity of tricuspid valve disease will become increasingly important for patient selection and treatment.

MULTIMODALITY IMAGING PLANNING FOR TRANSCATHETER TREATMENT OF THE TRICUSPID VALVE

In the United States, there are currently no commercially approved transcatheter therapies for use in tricuspid replacement or repair. Transcatheter interventions have been performed predominantly through compassionate, off-label use of devices targeting leaflet coaptation (Mitraclip, Abbott Vascular, Santa Clara, CA, USA) or implantation of a THV in a degenerated tricuspid ring or bioprosthesis (Edwards LifeSciences, Irvine, CA, USA).[1]

Because of the anterior location of the tricuspid valve, a combination of transesophageal echocardiography (TEE) and surface transthoracic echocardiography (TTE) have been used to assist in transcatheter plication of the tricuspid valve with the MitraClip.[9] However, with these ultrasound modalities, it is often difficult to discern adjacent anatomic landmarks and confidently identify which leaflets are visualized given the relative complex anatomy of the tricuspid valve. Combinations of preprocedural electrocardiography-gated cardiac computed tomography (CT), 3D printing, and 3D TEE have demonstrated to be useful in the intraprocedural visualization and planning of tricuspid interventions.[10]

MitraClip Implantation Within the Tricuspid Valve

Preprocedural imaging

Given the relative posterior location of the esophagus, traditional TEE views may not fully visualize the scope of tricuspid valve leaflets. When TEE has difficulty demonstrating the cause of the tricuspid regurgitation, a retrospectively gated CT scan is used to clearly identify leaflet motion, areas of malcoaptation, and commissure-to-commissure gap for clip anatomic suitability assessment (Fig. 1). Understanding the coaptation cause helps guide intraprocedural TEE imaging and probe manipulation.

Intraprocedural imaging

3D TEE plays an essential role in mapping the right atrium to guide catheter manipulation toward the tricuspid valve. 3D imaging of the tricuspid valve from the right atrium

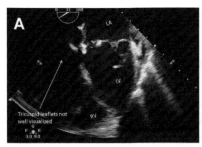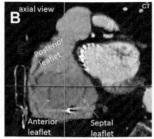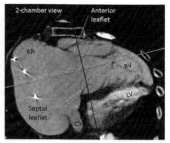

Posterior -> septal leaflet distance: 17.1mm
Anterior -> septal leaflet distance: 18.2mm

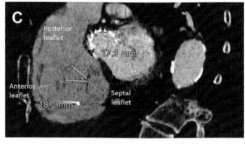

Fig. 1. Comparison of anatomic assessment of the tricuspid valve by TEE and multiplanar CT reconstruction. (*A*) 2D TEE imaging does not allow full visualization and identification of tricuspid leaflets with reproducible accuracy. (*B*) Retrospectively gated CT imaging of the tricuspid leaflets allow for identification of the three leaflet planes and (*C*) the commissure-to-commissure gaps between each leaflet.

into the right ventricle helps localize the mechanism of tricuspid regurgitation in the setting of pacer wire interaction. A large-sized field of view allows full visualization of the interatrial septum (medial), right atrium (lateral), and pacer wire (**Fig. 2**). Identification of a pacer wire at the anteroseptal commissure is more amenable to a tricuspid clip versus a pacer wire tapping the body of the septal leaflet open.

Unlike the traditional MitraClip approach to the mitral valve, the angulation of the tricuspid valve from the inferior vena cava (IVC) requires the delivery system to make sharp angulated turns in a smaller space. Hence, the operating team must be able to visualize when the system is tenting the interatrial septum (**Fig. 3**) and risk development of iatrogenic atrial septal defects or tenting the region of the coronary sinus. The latter is more commonly associated with development of complete heart block during tricuspid clip secondary to the location of the atrioventricular node in the triangle of Koch (see **Fig. 3**).

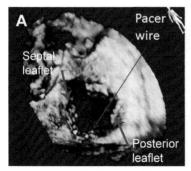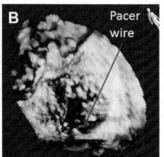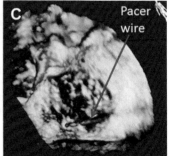

Fig. 2. 3D TEE visualization of the tricuspid leaflets from the right atrium. 3D *en face* visualization of the tricuspid leaflets clearly identifies where pacer wires interfere with leaflet coaptation. Panels (*A–C*) identify the pacer location and leaflet malcoaptation of the anterior and posterior tricuspid leaflets from diastole to systole (left to right).

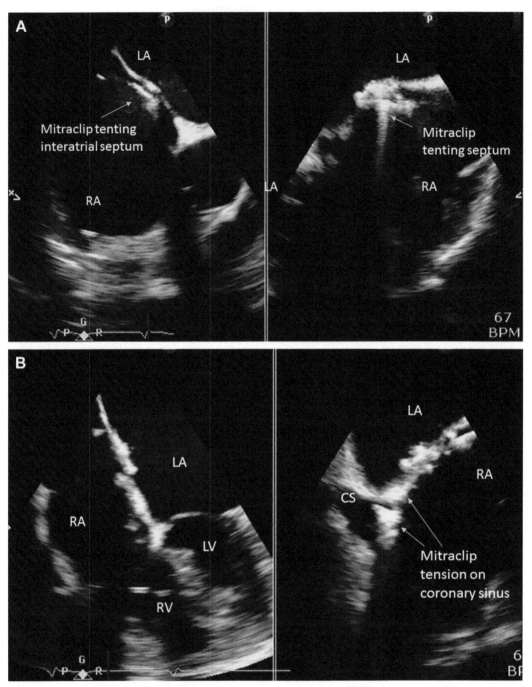

Fig. 3. Intraprocedural TEE tricuspid pearls. (A) Care must be taken to visualize the interatrial septum during navigation of the clip delivery system to the level of the tricuspid annulus to avoid unnecessary tenting of the interatrial septum. (B) Near the level of the tricuspid annulus, it is crucial to steer the delivery system and clip arms away from the triangle of Koch (region of coronary sinus) to avoid injury to the atrioventricular node, with resultant complete heart block. CS, coronary sinus; LA, left atrium; LV, left ventricle; RA, right atrium; RV, right ventricle.

COMPUTED TOMOGRAPHY PLANNING FOR TRICUSPID TRANSCATHETER HEART VALVE IN DEGENERATIVE SURGICAL RING/BIOPROSTHESIS

CT plays a crucial role in the planning of transcatheter tricuspid valve replacement (TTVR). Unlike the mitral annulus, the tricuspid annulus is 3D-shaped and surgical rings are not sutured into a planar surface. This makes deployment and landing of THV in the tricuspid position much more difficult (Fig. 4). Sizing of the tricuspid ring or bioprosthesis must be done in diastole when the valve is maximally open in a double-oblique 3D fashion to ensure all points of THV contact with the ring are accounted for (see Fig. 4). Fluoroscopic projections for THV delivery can then be mocked-up in an inverted overlay to allow maximal THV coaxiality alignment during valve deployment (see Fig. 4).

FUTURE CLINICAL DIRECTIONS
Imaging Techniques
Echocardiographic assessment of tricuspid valve severity is challenging and prone to high levels of interobserver variability and patient hemodynamic loading conditions at time of scan acquisition.[11] TTE is frequently limited in the visualization of the tricuspid valve leaflets. An understanding of which portions of the valve are abnormal is frequently made by inference based on traditional imaging conventions, not taking into patient-specific body habitus differences in valve orientation. CMR is advancing in the ability to assist in quantification of valvular heart disease when TTE imaging is insufficient.[12] Quantitative flow imaging has been applied in CMR to visualize the direction and severity of mitral and aortic regurgitation.[13,14] These same concepts may be applied to quantification of tricuspid regurgitation with potentially less interobserver variability (Fig. 5).

CMR may be of added value in understanding the structure and pathologies of the tricuspid valve. From a short axis stack of the tricuspid valve, cross-sectional imaging planes can be prescribed through each portion of individual tricuspid leaflets (Fig. 6). CMR-derived RV function has also been used to help with prognostication post-tricuspid valve surgery.[15] This volumetric approach may bring a more consummate analysis of the right ventricular function versus traditional single-plane 2D TTE evaluation utilizing tricuspid annular plane systolic

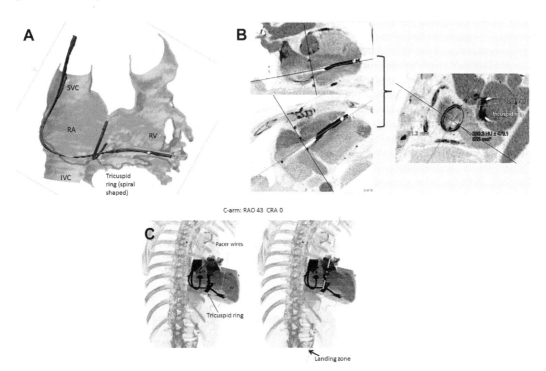

Fig. 4. CT planning for transcatheter tricuspid device implantation. (A) Computer-aided design analysis from CT imaging shows that the tricuspid ring is implanted on a nonplanar surface. (B) Double-oblique cut through the tricuspid annulus and ring during end-diastole allows for sizing of the landing zone for transcatheter heart valve implantation. (C) The angles for C-arm fluoroscopy that provide the optimal coaxiality during transcatheter tricuspid valve replacement deployment can be generated from CT.

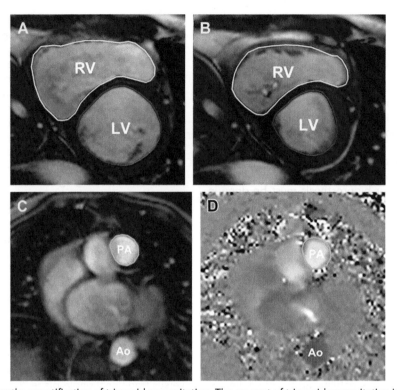

Fig. 5. CMR for the quantification of tricuspid regurgitation. The amount of tricuspid regurgitation is calculated as the difference between the total right ventricular stroke volume and forward flow through the pulmonary artery. The total right ventricular stroke volume is obtained by manual planimetry of the right ventricular endocardium in diastole (*A*) and systole (*B*). The forward flow through the pulmonary artery is obtained by using a quantitative velocity-encoded flow imaging. These images have a magnitude image for localization (*C*), as well as the actual velocity encoded flow image (*D*). On the flow images, the direction of flow is typically encoded with different intensities of black and white. Static tissue without flow is in gray.

excursion.[16–18] CMR also provides valuable information regarding other contributors to valve disease. Steady state free progression (SSFP) images are used to interrogate chordal attachments and wall motion abnormalities. Myocardial tissue characteristics, such as tissue scar or fibrosis, are evaluated using late gadolinium-enhanced images (LGE). LGE and other tissue characterization sequences available for CMR are helpful to identify if a cardiac mass may be the cause of an underlying mechanism for tricuspid valve disease.[19,20]

FUTURE THERAPIES

Caval Valve Implantation

In the setting of severe tricuspid regurgitation, many times the tricuspid annulus has dilated to sizes exceeding the ability of a clip to grasp opposing leaflets. In the absence of a commercially available transcatheter tricuspid replacement valve or annular solution, the concept of caval valve implantation (CAVI) is being actively studied.[10] Heterotopic implantation of a valve in the IVC and superior vena cava (SVC) has

been demonstrated to help redirect the tricuspid regurgitant jet away from the hepatic venous system. Accurate sizing of the right atrium-IVC junction is important in valve size selection. Contrast-enhanced retrospectively gated CT is used to size the specified landing zone in end-systole. 3D CT also allows visualization of the depth of the IVC tubular landing zone to ensure there is no blockage of flow to the most superior hepatic vein post-CAVI implantation. Early case reports demonstrate improvement in patients' right-sided heart failure symptoms of congestion post-CAVI.[10]

The novelty of CAVI resides in the ease of deployment of a heterotopic device in the IVC.[21] In addition, implantation of a CAVI device does not anatomically preclude patients from future tricuspid annular or leaflet therapies. CAVI is currently being prospectively studied as part of the HOVER (Heterotopic Implantation of the Edwards Sapien Transcatheter Valve in the Inferior Vena Cava for the Treatment of Severe Tricuspid Regurgitation) study in the United States (ClinicalTrials.gov identifier,

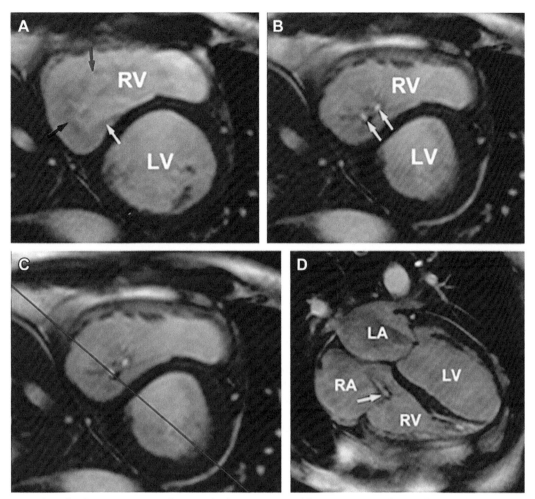

Fig. 6. CMR for the interrogation of tricuspid valve structure and function. (A) Steady state free progression (SSFP) cine still frame showing short axis of the left and right ventricle in diastole with focus on tricuspid valve morphology. Septal leaflet is indicated by the yellow arrow, the posterior leaflet by the blue arrow, and the anterior leaflet by the red arrow. (B) SSFP-focused view of the tricuspid valve in systole. Yellow arrows demonstrate two regions of incomplete coaptation at the leaflet tips. This image could be used to measure an anatomic regurgitant orifice area by planimetry. (C) CMR is not limited by imaging planes, and the red line shows the prescribing of a future imaging plane that optimizes the center of the jet of tricuspid regurgitation. (D) Resulting SSFP cine image obtained from the prior prescribed red line. Yellow arrow indicates the jet of regurgitation. LA, left atrium; LV, left ventricle; RA, right atrium; RV, right ventricle.

NCT02339974) and the TRICAVAL (Treatment of Severe Secondary Tricuspid Regurgitation in Patients With Advance Heart Failure with Caval Valve Implantation of the Edwards Sapien XT Valve) study in Germany (ClinicalTrials.gov identifier, NCT02387697).[21]

SUMMARY

There is increasing awareness of the prevalence of tricuspid valve disease.[1] However, imaging techniques and commercial availability of transcatheter devices for tricuspid interventions is lagging behind the speed of development of new aortic and mitral THV therapies. Once the forgotten valve, the tricuspid anatomy has proved to be more variable than traditional aortic or mitral landing zones. To ensure the success of advancing transcatheter tricuspid therapies, further research into imaging techniques and development of tricuspid annular solutions will no doubt be necessary to push therapy development forward.

REFERENCES

1. Vahanian A. Transcatheter tricuspid intervention: the new challenge of structural valve intervention. EuroIntervention 2018;13(14):1631–3.

2. Lamers WH, Viragh S, Wessels A, et al. Formation of the tricuspid valve in the human heart. Circulation 1995;91(1):111–21.

3. Silver MD, Lam JH, Ranganathan N, et al. Morphology of the human tricuspid valve. Circulation 1971;43(3):333–48.

4. Wafae N, Hayashi H, Gerola LR, et al. Anatomical study of the human tricuspid valve. Surg Radiol Anat 1990;12(1):37–41.

5. Sutton JP 3rd, Ho SY, Vogel M, et al. Is the morphologically right atrioventricular valve tricuspid? J Heart Valve Dis 1995;4(6):571–5.

6. Athavale S, Deopujari R, Sinha U, et al. Is tricuspid valve really tricuspid? Anat Cell Biol 2017;50(1):1–6.

7. Nath J, Foster E, Heidenreich PA. Impact of tricuspid regurgitation on long-term survival. J Am Coll Cardiol 2004;43(3):405–9.

8. Sadeghpour A, Hassanzadeh M, Kyavar M, et al. Impact of severe tricuspid regurgitation on long term survival. Res Cardiovasc Med 2013;2(3): 121–6.

9. Khalique OK, Hahn RT. Role of echocardiography in transcatheter valvular heart disease interventions. Curr Cardiol Rep 2017;19(12):128.

10. O'Neill B, Wang DD, Pantelic M, et al. Transcatheter caval valve implantation using multimodality imaging: roles of TEE, CT, and 3D printing. JACC Cardiovasc Imaging 2015;8(2):221–5.

11. Grant AD, Thavendiranathan P, Rodriguez LL, et al. Development of a consensus algorithm to improve interobserver agreement and accuracy in the determination of tricuspid regurgitation severity. J Am Soc Echocardiogr 2014;27(3):277–84.

12. Zoghbi WA, Adams D, Bonow RO, et al. Recommendations for noninvasive evaluation of native valvular regurgitation: a report from the American society of echocardiography developed in collaboration with the society for cardiovascular magnetic resonance. J Am Soc Echocardiogr 2017;30(4): 303–71.

13. Lee JC, Branch KR, Hamilton-Craig C, et al. Evaluation of aortic regurgitation with cardiac magnetic resonance imaging: a systematic review. Heart 2018;104(2):103–10.

14. Krieger EV, Lee J, Branch KR, et al. Quantitation of mitral regurgitation with cardiac magnetic resonance imaging: a systematic review. Heart 2016; 102(23):1864–70.

15. Park JB, Kim HK, Jung JH, et al. Prognostic value of cardiac MR imaging for preoperative assessment of patients with severe functional tricuspid regurgitation. Radiology 2016;280(3):723–34.

16. Corona-Villalobos CP, Kamel IR, Rastegar N, et al. Bidimensional measurements of right ventricular function for prediction of survival in patients with pulmonary hypertension: comparison of reproducibility and time of analysis with volumetric cardiac magnetic resonance imaging analysis. Pulm Circ 2015;5(3):527–37.

17. Lee JZ, Low SW, Pasha AK, et al. Comparison of tricuspid annular plane systolic excursion with fractional area change for the evaluation of right ventricular systolic function: a meta-analysis. Open Heart 2018;5(1):e000667.

18. Soslow JH, Usoro E, Wang L, et al. Evaluation of tricuspid annular plane systolic excursion measured with cardiac MRI in children with tetralogy of Fallot. Cardiol Young 2016;26(4):718–24.

19. Fang L, He L, Chen Y, et al. Infiltrating lipoma of the right ventricle involving the interventricular septum and tricuspid valve: report of a rare case and literature review. Medicine (Baltimore) 2016;95(3):e2561.

20. Srivatsa SV, Adhikari P, Chaudhry P, et al. Multimodality imaging of right-sided (tricuspid valve) papillary fibroelastoma: recognition of a surgically remediable disease. Case Rep Oncol 2013;6(3): 485–9.

21. O'Neill BP. Caval valve implantation: are 2 valves better than 1? Circ Cardiovasc Interv 2018;11(2): e006334.

Identification and Quantification of Degenerative and Functional Mitral Regurgitation for Patient Selection for Transcatheter Mitral Valve Repair

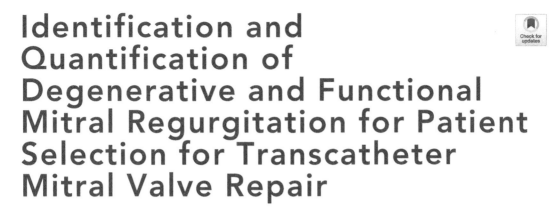

Tiffany Chen, MD[a], Victor A. Ferrari, MD[b,c],
Frank E. Silvestry, MD[d],*

KEYWORDS

- Mitral regurgitation • Transcatheter mitral valve repair • Echocardiography
- Mitral valve prolapse • Cardiac imaging • MitraClip

KEY POINTS

- Mitral regurgitation (MR) can be due to valvular degeneration, secondary to ventricular remodeling, or a combination of the 2 mechanisms.
- Edge-to-edge leaflet repair is the only approved transcatheter mitral valve repair technique in the United States; novel approaches targeting different components of the mitral anatomy are emerging.
- Imaging with echocardiography establishes the cause of MR, determines anatomic feasibility of transcatheter repair, and grades the severity of MR.
- Feasibility of MitraClip edge-to-edge repair requires sufficient leaflet tissue for capture, leaflet motion that is not excessively restricted or redundant, and central MR origin.
- Quantification of MR involves integration of various echocardiographic (including 3-dimensional–derived) parameters and potentially advanced imaging with cardiac magnetic resonance to resolve discrepancies.

 Video content accompanies this article at http://www.interventional.theclinics.com.

INTRODUCTION

Chronic mitral regurgitation (MR) is prevalent in the adult population and leads to significant morbidity and mortality.[1–5] Moderate or severe MR affects an estimated 1.7% of the adult population in the United States, more than 4-fold higher than aortic stenosis.[1] Although mitral valve surgery has been the mainstay of treatment of symptomatic severe degenerative mitral regurgitation (DMR), many patients at high or prohibitive

---

Disclosure Statement: F.E. Silvestry is a site sub-investigator for Edwards CardiaQ and CardioBand. No disclosures for the remaining authors.
^a Department of Medicine, Cardiovascular Division, University of Pennsylvania, 11-134 South PCAM, 3400 Civic Center Boulevard, Philadelphia, PA 19104, USA; ^b Department of Medicine, Cardiovascular Division, University of Pennsylvania, 11-136 South PCAM, 3400 Civic Center Boulevard, Philadelphia, PA 19104, USA; ^c Department of Radiology, University of Pennsylvania, 11-136 South PCAM, 3400 Civic Center Boulevard, Philadelphia, PA, USA; ^d Department of Medicine, Cardiovascular Division, University of Pennsylvania, 11-133 South PCAM, 3400 Civic Center Boulevard, Philadelphia, PA 19104, USA
* Corresponding author.
E-mail address: fsilvest@pennmedicine.upenn.edu

Intervent Cardiol Clin 7 (2018) 387–404
https://doi.org/10.1016/j.iccl.2018.04.002
2211-7458/18/© 2018 Elsevier Inc. All rights reserved.

operative risk are now referred for consideration of percutaneous mitral valve repair. Imaging, primarily with echocardiography, plays a crucial role in the characterization and quantification of MR to determine candidacy for transcatheter mitral valve repair.

CAUSE AND PATHOPHYSIOLOGY OF MITRAL REGURGITATION

MR can result from several mechanisms, which are broadly characterized into either a primary abnormality of the valvular apparatus or a secondary dysfunction due to other cardiac disease.

Primary Mitral Regurgitation

The most common cause of primary MR is degenerative disease, whether due to fibroelastic deficiency (FED) or myxomatous infiltration (Barlow disease). The former is associated with focal leaflet involvement, whereas the latter manifests as myxoid degeneration of the valve with diffuse thickening and multisegment redundancy. FED is characterized by a lack of connective tissue resulting in leaflet and chordal thinning and eventual chordal rupture manifesting as prolapse or flail of a single leaflet segment. Barlow disease results in marked leaflet thickening, large redundant leaflets, chordal elongation or rupture, and annular dilatation. Patients with Barlow disease generally have complex valve pathologic condition and dysfunction, which is most often multisegmental. A forme fruste phenotype of Barlow disease may present with intermediate features. Mitral valve prolapse can ultimately progress to leaflet flail, which is nearly uniformly associated with severe MR and chordal rupture.[2,6,7]

Causes of primary mitral regurgitation
Fibroelastic deficiency
Myxomatous infiltration
Rheumatic disease
Infective or nonbacterial thrombotic endocarditis
Mitral annular calcification
Radiation heart disease
Congenital malformations

Functional Mitral Regurgitation

In contrast to primary MR, functional mitral regurgitation (FMR) is associated with relatively normal mitral leaflet structure and is typically attributed to myocardial pathologic condition.

Left ventricular remodeling, whether due to ischemic injury or other cardiomyopathy, causes apical and outward displacement of the papillary muscle or muscles leading to restriction and tethering of the mitral valve leaflets.[8] MR results because of imbalance between the opposing tethering and closing forces that drive leaflet coaptation. Distortion of mitral annular geometry further perpetuates MR, as the normally saddle-shaped annulus dilates and flattens.[9,10] Less commonly, FMR may also result from isolated annular dilatation due to severe left atrial (LA) enlargement such as in chronic atrial fibrillation or restrictive cardiomyopathy.[11]

Carpentier Classification

Mitral valve dysfunction can also be categorized according to leaflet motion with the Carpentier classification system (Fig. 1), which originated as a framework for determining an approach to surgical repair.[12] Type I dysfunction is associated with normal leaflet motion, such as in atrial FMR or leaflet perforation. Type II describes excessive leaflet motion, which occurs with mitral valve prolapse and leaflet flail. Type III dysfunction refers to restricted leaflet motion and is subdivided into type IIIa (diastolic and systolic restriction) and type IIIb (systolic restriction). Rheumatic, carcinoid, radiation heart disease, and other inflammatory conditions that restrict mitral valve opening are classified as Carpentier type IIIa. FMR due to ventricular dilatation and ischemic MR causes type IIIb dysfunction (restricted mitral valve closure).

Hemodynamic Effects of Chronic Mitral Regurgitation

Regardless of the cause or mechanism, chronic MR creates an additional volume load on the left ventricle (LV), which responds with eccentric hypertrophy. In the compensated phase of chronic severe MR, total stroke volume increases proportional to the increased preload, thus allowing LV ejection fraction (LVEF) to remain greater than normal. As myocardial dysfunction, cell death, and myocardial fibrosis develop, ventricular stroke volume diminishes, and LVEF will decline. Other hemodynamic effects of chronic severe MR include increased LA pressure and consequent pulmonary venous hypertension. Associated LA remodeling and dilation may also result in eventual atrial fibrillation.

TRANSCATHETER MITRAL VALVE REPAIR

MR is more prevalent in the elderly, nearly 10% of Americans older than 75 years of age have

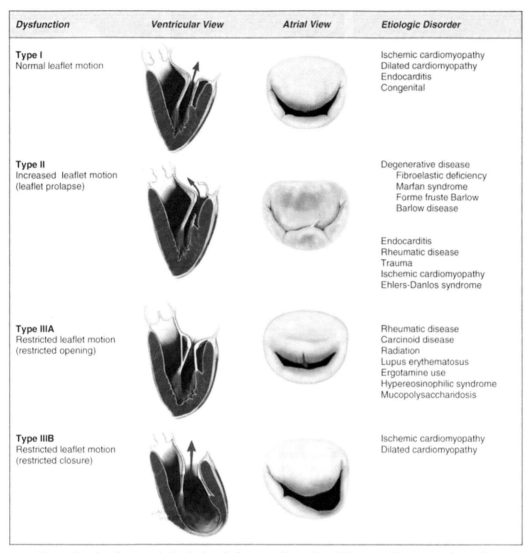

Dysfunction	Ventricular View	Atrial View	Etiologic Disorder
Type I Normal leaflet motion			Ischemic cardiomyopathy Dilated cardiomyopathy Endocarditis Congenital

Type II
Increased leaflet motion
(leaflet prolapse)
			Degenerative disease
			  Fibroelastic deficiency
			  Marfan syndrome
			  Forme fruste Barlow
			  Barlow disease
			
			Endocarditis
			Rheumatic disease
			Trauma
			Ischemic cardiomyopathy
			Ehlers-Danlos syndrome

Type IIIA Restricted leaflet motion (restricted opening)			Rheumatic disease Carcinoid disease Radiation Lupus erythematosus Ergotamine use Hypereosinophilic syndrome Mucopolysaccharidosis
Type IIIB Restricted leaflet motion (restricted closure)			Ischemic cardiomyopathy Dilated cardiomyopathy

Fig. 1. Carpentier classification of mitral valve dysfunction. (*From* Otto CM, Bonow RO. Valvular heart disease. In: Mann DL, Zipes DP, Libby P, et al, editors. Braunwald's heart disease: a textbook of cardiovascular medicine. 10th edition. Philadelphia: Elsevier; 2015. p. 1480; with permission.)

moderate or severe MR.[1] They are also often at high or prohibitive risk for mitral valve surgery due to comorbidities. Transcatheter therapies have thus emerged as an attractive alternative to surgery for these individuals, particularly as the general population ages.

Edge-to-Edge Leaflet Repair

Currently, the only transcatheter mitral valve repair system approved by the US Food and Drug Administration is the MitraClip (Abbott Vascular, Santa Clara, CA, USA). Edge-to-edge leaflet coaptation with the MitraClip device results in a double orifice mitral valve, similar to the Alfieri technique for surgical repair

(Fig. 2).[13] The efficacy and safety of the MitraClip system were demonstrated by the ndovascular Valve Edge-to-Edge Repair (EVEREST) II randomized control trial, in which patients with severe MR (predominantly degenerative) had fewer adverse cardiovascular events and similar mortality with the MitraClip as compared with mitral valve surgery but less reduction in MR.[14,15] MitraClip therapy has been associated with reduction in MR, improvement in symptoms, and signs of reverse LV remodeling in patients at high or prohibitive surgical risk (defined as ≥8% predicted risk of mortality for surgical mitral valve replacement by the Society of Thoracic Surgery score, or the presence of other

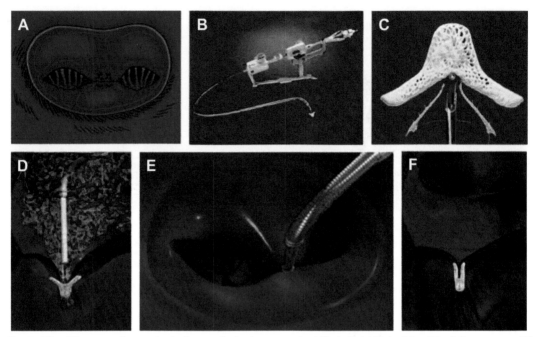

Fig. 2. MitraClip transcatheter mitral valve repair. Analogous to the Alfieri stitch (*A*), the MitraClip delivery system (*B*) accomplishes edge-to-edge repair by deploying a clip device (*C*) at the center of the coaptation line (*D–F*). (*From* Herrmann HC. Transcatheter mitral valve repair and replacement. In: Otto CM, Bonow RO, editors. Valvular heart disease: a companion to Braunwald's heart disease. 4th edition. Philadelphia: Elsevier; 2014. p. 342; with permission.)

comorbidities, such as porcelain aorta, hostile chest, frailty, advanced liver disease, or severe pulmonary hypertension).[16,17] Thus, the MitraClip is approved in the United States for treatment of severe, symptomatic primary MR in patients at prohibitive risk for mitral valve surgery.

Other Techniques

Numerous transcatheter mitral valve repair devices other than the MitraClip edge-to-edge repair system have been developed and are currently under clinical investigation. Each transcatheter repair technique addresses a singular component of the mitral valve complex that results in MR: the leaflets (as in the MitraClip), the mitral annulus (either directly or indirectly via the coronary sinus),[18–20] chordae,[21,22] or the LV. Therefore, anatomic considerations for suitability of transcatheter repair are individualized for each device. Another emerging therapeutic option is transcatheter mitral valve replacement, which relies heavily on multimodality imaging for preprocedural planning.[23,24]

ECHOCARDIOGRAPHIC ASSESSMENT OF MITRAL REGURGITATION

General Considerations

Assessment with echocardiography is essential to patient selection for transcatheter mitral

valve repair in several ways. First, the presence of MR and its underlying mechanism can be established. Second, the anatomy of the mitral valve apparatus as it relates to the feasibility of the specific repair technique can be evaluated. Finally, the severity of MR can be quantified. Candidacy for transcatheter mitral valve repair is a nuanced decision dependent on a comprehensive patient evaluation encompassing all these factors, in addition to clinical context.[25–27]

Determining whether the mechanism of MR is primary or secondary is pivotal, because management strategies differ and the role of transcatheter therapy for the latter remains unclear and under current investigation. Although numerous studies have failed to show a survival benefit to mitral valve surgery for FMR, symptom relief and reduction in heart failure have been observed.[28,29] The ongoing COAPT (Clinical Outcomes Assessment of the MitraClip Percutaneous Therapy for High Risk Surgical Patients) trial is designed to assess whether transcatheter repair with the MitraClip also achieves improvement in symptoms and reduction in heart failure hospitalization (clinicaltrials.gov, NCT01626079). Presently, the MitraClip has approval in the United States for primary MR only, whereas it is approved for both primary and secondary MR in Europe.

Transthoracic echocardiography (TTE) is typically sufficient for distinguishing primary from secondary MR. Components of the mitral apparatus, as well as left ventricular size and function, are readily evaluated by TTE. High-temporal resolution makes assessment of leaflet motion (and determination of Carpentier class) possible. Transesophageal echocardiography (TEE) allows for visualization of the mitral valve in multiple imaging planes with higher spatial resolution to better localize valvular pathologic condition. Three-dimensional echocardiography (3DE) further enhances visualization of the mitral valve with the ability to produce additional perspectives, such as the en face surgeon's view, and reconstructions of the complex geometry of the mitral annulus and leaflets.[30] Although more detailed anatomic assessment can be accomplished by TEE, procedural sedation alters loading conditions and may underestimate MR severity.

Degenerative Mitral Regurgitation

DMR is characterized by mitral valve prolapse, defined as excursion of more than 2 mm beyond the annular plane during systole in the parasternal long-axis view, which transects the mitral valve at the most basal points of the saddle-shaped mitral annulus at A2/P2 (**Fig. 3**). Because of the shape of the mitral annulus, apparent prolapse in alternate views may be misleading. FED involves isolated segmental prolapse, most commonly of the P2 scallop, and may be associated with chordal rupture leading to a flail segment (**Fig. 4**, Video 1). In contrast, diffuse leaflet thickening with multisegmental prolapse and chordal elongation is characteristic of Barlow disease (**Fig. 5**, Video 2). In addition, calcification of the annulus and subvalvular apparatus is more frequent with Barlow disease.[31] The mitral annulus also dilates more severely in Barlow disease, particularly in the intercommissural dimension, although dynamicity throughout the cardiac cycle is retained.[32] 3DE is instrumental in localization of prolapsed and flail segments of the mitral valve. Furthermore, measurements of billowing height and volume by 3DE have been shown to differentiate between the spectrum of degenerative mitral valve disease and normal anatomy.[33] DMR typically

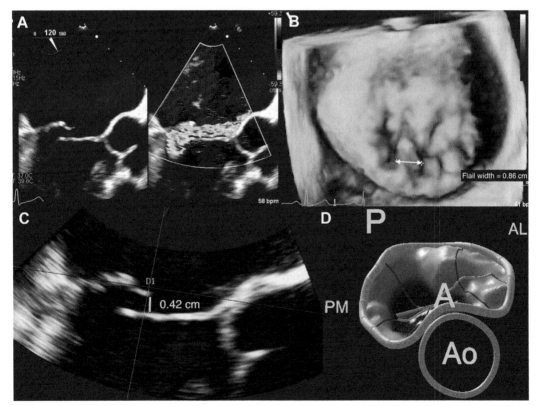

Fig. 3. DMR. (*A*) Posterior leaflet flail resulting in eccentric MR directed anteriorly. (*B*) 3D TEE en face view of mitral valve localizes flail segment to P2. Flail width measures 0.86 cm. (*C*) Flail gap measures 0.42 cm, obtained from 3D multiplanar reconstruction. (*D*) 3D parametric map of myxomatous mitral valve with predominant P1 prolapse. A, anterior; AL, anterolateral; Ao, aorta; P, posterior; PM, posteromedial.

A　　　　　　　　　　　　　　**B**

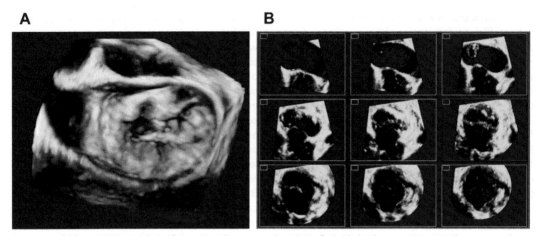

Fig. 4. P3 flail on 3D TEE. (A) En face view showing isolated P3 flail, likely due to FED. (B) Short-axis "slices" through the mitral valve from LA to LV, oriented with posterior annulus on top. Flail segment at P3 is visualized in the top right panel with subsequent panels showing posterior leaflet prolapse.

occurs in mid-late systole, when mal-coaptation due to leaflet redundancy is greatest. The regurgitant jet of focal prolapse or flail is often eccentric and directed toward the opposing leaflet, which may complicate quantification (Video 3). Diffuse leaflet redundancy in Barlow disease may result in multiple, complex regurgitant jets, also complicating quantification.

Functional Mitral Regurgitation

Echocardiographic features of FMR include altered ventricular morphology and function as well as the resultant distortion in mitral annular geometry and leaflet motion. Not only is LV systolic function severely impaired but also indications of adverse remodeling are typically present, such as chamber dilatation and increased sphericity. Because LV dilatation may be either the cause or the consequence of MR, careful assessment of the mitral apparatus by echocardiography is especially important for distinguishing FMR from a primary cause. In FMR, leaflet tenting due to apical displacement of the papillary muscles may be best visualized on TTE from the apical 4-chamber view. The distance from leaflet tips to the annular plane is known as the coaptation depth (or height), which is increased in FMR (Fig. 6A, Video 4). The degree of apical tethering can also be quantified by measuring the tenting area formed by the leaflet tips and the annular plane (Fig. 6D), or a tenting volume with 3DE.[34] Both these parameters have some correlation with the severity of FMR.[35] Annular changes associated with FMR include dilatation, flattening of the saddle shape, and loss of dynamicity throughout the cardiac cycle.[9,10] Dilatation tends to affect the posterior annulus

predominantly and in the septal-lateral dimension, as opposed to the intercommissural dimension that is more affected by Barlow disease (Fig. 7).[36]

Although apical tethering can result from any dilated cardiomyopathy, ischemic cardiomyopathy with infarction of the inferior and inferolateral walls is particularly susceptible because of the location of the papillary muscles. Thus, ischemic MR is a common form of FMR. Inferior myocardial infarction is associated with an asymmetric tethering pattern in which the posterior mitral leaflet (especially at P3) is more restricted than the anterior, resulting in one or more posteriorly directed MR jets.[37] The anterior leaflet can develop a bend, because of restriction of its midsection by strut secondary chords, forming a "seagull" or "hockey-stick" appearance (Fig. 6B, Video 5). Unlike in rheumatic mitral disease, diastolic doming and commissural fusion are absent. Anterior leaflet override from asymmetric tethering may also be misinterpreted as mitral valve prolapse. In contrast to DMR, the timing of FMR is typically holosystolic in which there is a biphasic pattern with slight reduction in MR in midsystole when the closing force opposing tethering is greatest.[38] Although these characteristic features help differentiate degenerative from FMR (Table 1), a mixed cause may be present and must also be considered.

Anatomic Considerations for Transcatheter Repair

Because each transcatheter repair technique targets a single component of the mitral valve complex, the pathologic anatomy mediating MR has significant implications for the likelihood of

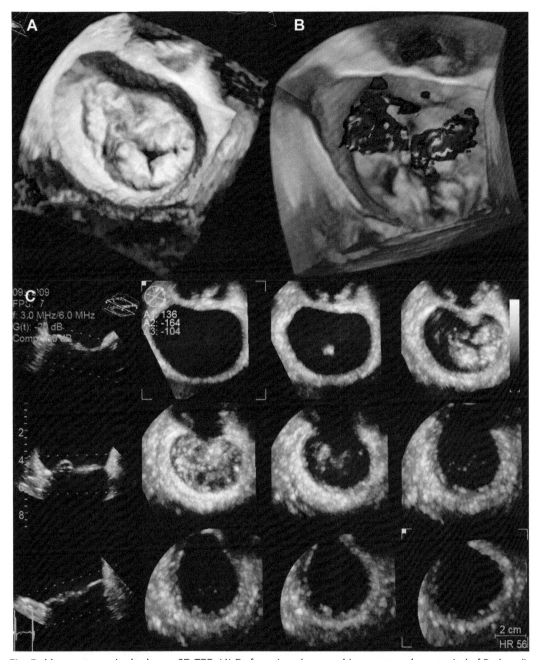

Fig. 5. Myxomatous mitral valve on 3D TEE. (*A*) En face view shows multisegment prolapse typical of Barlow disease, and P2 flail. (*B*) 3D color Doppler shows MR originating centrally at the flail segment. (*C*) Serial short-axis "slices" through the mitral valve from LA to LV showing the flail segment in the top center panel as well as bileaflet prolapse and thickening.

successful repair with each technique. Careful morphologic assessment of the mitral valve is performed primarily with TEE, although there is an emerging role for computed tomography (CT) imaging for certain repair techniques. For example, evaluating the relationship of the coronary sinus to the mitral annulus and the left circumflex artery by CT is important for indirect annuloplasty planning. Annular size and calcification are also readily assessed by CT. CT has become invaluable for transcatheter mitral valve replacement as well.

For edge-to-edge coaptation with the Mitra-Clip device, specific anatomic features have

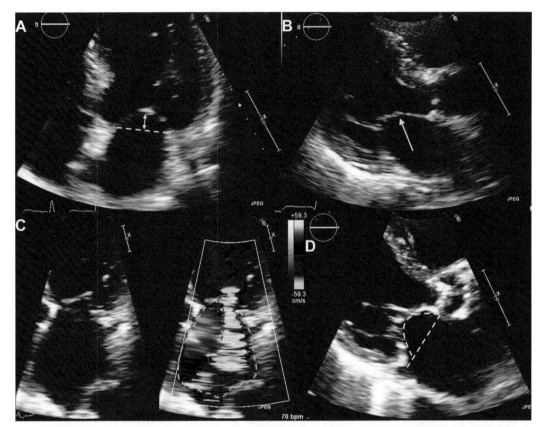

Fig. 6. FMR on TTE. (A) Increased coaptation depth due to apical tethering of mitral leaflets. (B) Anterior leaflet "hockey-stick" bend (*arrow*) due to tethering. (C) MR secondary to posterior leaflet restriction. Jet area (*traced in red*) is close to 40% of the LA area (*traced in green*), suggesting significant MR. (D) Apical tethering due to ischemic cardiomyopathy increases tenting area (*outlined in yellow*).

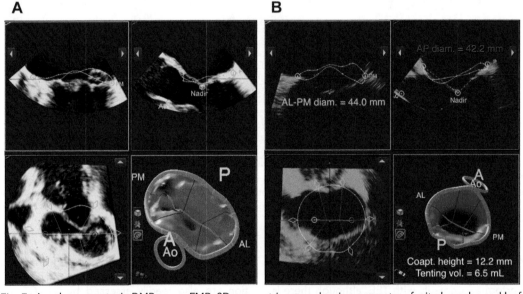

Fig. 7. Annular geometry in DMR versus FMR. 3D parametric maps showing geometry of mitral annulus and leaflets. (A) DMR from Barlow disease with multisegment prolapse, mostly at P3, and annular dilation predominantly in the IC dimension. (B) FMR with annular dilation with increased IC (AL-PM) and AP (S-L) diameters of greater than 40 mm. Apical tethering results in increased coaptation height (depth) of 12 mm and tenting volume of 6.5 mL. AL-PM, anterolateral-posteromedial; AP, anterior-posterior; IC, intercommissural; S-L, septal-lateral.

Table 1
Echocardiographic features of degenerative mitral regurgitation and functional mitral regurgitation

	DMR	FMR
Leaflet structure	Thickened, focal, or diffuse	Normal or minimally thickened
Leaflet motion	Prolapse ± flail	Restricted/tethered, anterior leaflet override
LV morphology	Normal or minimally dilated	Severely dilated, spherical
Papillary muscles	Normal	Apically displaced
Chordae	Elongated ± rupture	Tethered
Coaptation depth	Normal	Increased
Tenting volume/area	Normal	Increased
MR timing	Mid-late systolic or holosystolic	Holosystolic, biphasic
MR jet direction	Eccentric, wall-impinging, opposite prolapsed segment	Less eccentric, toward tethered leaflet
Annulus	Dilated (IC > SL), flattened	Dilated (SL > IC), flattened, adynamic
ERO	Circular	Elliptical, crescentic

Abbreviations: IC, intercommissural; SL, septal-lateral.

been identified to be favorable for procedural success (Table 2). In order to facilitate leaflet capture, there must be (1) sufficient leaflet tissue without significant calcification, (2) leaflet motion that is neither too restricted nor too excessive, and (3) sufficient leaflet length. Infective endocarditis, leaflet perforation, and cleft are generally contraindications to the procedure. Rheumatic heart disease is another contraindication due to the risk of reducing the mitral valve area and worsening mitral stenosis. Mitra-Clip is associated with an approximately 40% reduction in mitral valve area from baseline.[39] Therefore, mitral valve area less than 4.0 cm^2 was an exclusion criterion for the EVEREST trials.[40] Direct planimetry of the mitral valve area can be accurately obtained by 3DE and should

Table 2
Anatomic features favorable for MitraClip

Mitral valve area ≥4 cm^2

Central origin of MR at A2/P2

DMR:	FMR:
Flail gap <10 mm	Coaptation length
Flail width <15 mm	≥2 mm
	Coaptation depth
	≤11 mm

Minimal calcification of grasping zone and annulus

Minimal annular dilatation

Absence of rheumatic disease, leaflet perforation, cleft

be performed routinely.[25] The EVEREST trial used anatomic inclusions for DMR and FMR based on prediction of system performance with specific anatomy and thus are informative but are by no means absolute. Real world, post-marketing experience (especially outside the United States) with MitraClip has proven that EVEREST inclusion and exclusion criteria are not absolute but remain a reasonable starting point. Anatomic inclusion criteria for EVEREST were flail gap less than 10 mm, flail width less than 15 mm, coaptation depth ≤11 mm, and coaptation length ≥2 mm.[40] Severe, multisegment prolapse presents a challenge for leaflet capture and effective reduction in leaflet billowing. Approximation of the leaflets is also difficult in the presence of severe tethering of the anatomically shorter posterior leaflet and profound annular dilatation. Furthermore, MR predominantly arising from A2/P2 is favorable because of the lower risk of entanglement in the chordae during clip delivery at this region of the leaflet rough zone, where chordal attachments are fewest. The ideal grasping zone is thus near the center of the coaptation line. Significant calcification in the grasping zone increases the risk of leaflet perforation or clip detachment and should be excluded.[41,42]

All these morphologic characteristics contribute to the likelihood of successful Mitra-Clip repair, but they do not represent absolute criteria. As experience with transcatheter edge-to-edge repair and three-dimensional (3D) TEE imaging guidance increases, the anatomic eligibility for MitraClip has expanded beyond the EVEREST echocardiographic criteria.[43,44] For instance, successful MitraClip repair has been described in patients with failed annuloplasty rings.[45,46] Some proposed strategies to facilitate leaflet capture in challenging scenarios include approaching from an acute angle for extreme flail, rapid pacing when coaptation is more favorable during systole, administering adenosine when coaptation is more favorable in diastole, and stepwise approximation with successive clips.[47]

QUANTIFICATION OF MITRAL REGURGITATION

In addition to establishing the mechanism of MR and assessing mitral anatomy, determining MR severity is another key component of the evaluation for transcatheter mitral repair. Mitral repair is generally indicated for severe MR (3+ or 4+). Quantification of MR can be complicated, because of its dynamicity and susceptibility to the influence of hemodynamic loading conditions. An integrative approach is recommended to most accurately grade MR severity, given the individual limitations of each of the quantitative parameters.[26,48] Thus, the echocardiographic evaluation should be comprehensive in assessing MR severity. In broad terms, echocardiographic methods for grading MR severity can be categorized into the following:

Methods for grading mitral regurgitation severity by echocardiography
• Semiquantitative measures (Doppler)
• Quantitative parameters (proximal flow convergence)
• Volumetric methods
• Indirect and/or supportive signs

Furthermore, there is increasing evidence for MR quantitation with 3D TEE methods.[49–51] Although TTE is often the initial imaging modality for MR quantification, further investigation with TEE or cardiac magnetic resonance (CMR) imaging should be pursued in situations of uncertainty or suboptimal image quality. TTE and CMR avoid sedation that can alter loading conditions and are therefore preferred to TEE for assessment of MR severity.

Semiquantitative Methods
Detection by color flow Doppler is often the initial indication of MR. Visual assessment of the regurgitant jet area by color Doppler offers a quick but imprecise measure of MR severity. The proportion of the LA area occupied by the regurgitant color flow jet, as imaged from an apical window (Fig. 6C), has some correlation to MR severity. A jet area of less than 20% generally corresponds to mild MR, whereas a ratio of greater than 40% usually indicates severe MR.[25,52] However, visual assessment by color Doppler is insufficient for grading MR severity because of variability due to instrument settings and hemodynamic conditions.[48] Lowering the Nyquist limit (aliasing velocity) or increasing gain settings can accentuate the apparent severity of MR by color Doppler. Systemic hypertension increases the transmitral pressure gradient and thus the momentum of the regurgitant jet, increasing the apparent severity by Doppler. Conversely, in acute torrential MR, severity by color Doppler may be underestimated because of low-velocity regurgitant flow resulting from early equilibration of LA and LV pressures. In addition, LA size and compliance can affect the appearance of MR by color Doppler. Characteristics of the MR jet itself also influence its apparent severity by color Doppler jet area. Asymmetric jets with noncircular regurgitant orifices can have variable jet areas, depending on the 2-dimensional (2D) imaging plane. The severity of eccentric jets is prone to underestimation with the jet area method for several reasons. First, wall-impinged eccentric jets tend to course along the LA wall (Coanda effect) while spreading out laterally, such that jet size may appear smaller in the imaging plane. Second, impingement from the LA wall prevents entrainment of blood on all sides of the MR jet, thus reducing the apparent severity by jet area.[53,54] Because jet area is estimated from a single systolic frame, dynamic and nonholosystolic MR jets are also difficult to assess with this method.

Continuous-wave (CW) Doppler offers a qualitative method to evaluate MR severity and is particularly useful for assessing temporal variation in MR. Similar to the jet area method by color Doppler, assessment of MR by the CW Doppler spectral recording is simple to perform and is reliant on alignment of the ultrasound beam with the MR jet. Spectral density is proportional to the number of red blood cells reflecting the Doppler signal and thus is an indirect measure of regurgitant volume (RVol). CW Doppler signal density similar to that of antegrade flow generally indicates moderate-severe MR.[55] In addition, CW Doppler delineates the timing and duration of MR within the cardiac cycle. Non-holosystolic MR, such as late-systolic MR associated with mitral valve prolapse, is rarely severe.[56] In acute severe MR, the CW Doppler tracing has a characteristic triangular shape with early peaking at a low maximal velocity.

A semiquantitative parameter derived from 2D color Doppler that is less dependent on flow rate and hemodynamic loading conditions is the vena contracta width (VCW). The vena contracta is the narrowest portion of the MR jet with the highest-velocity laminar flow and located at or immediately downstream of the anatomic regurgitant orifice. The cross-sectional area of the vena contracta forms the effective regurgitant orifice area (EROA), of which the VCW is a linear surrogate. Measurement of the VCW should be performed in an imaging plane perpendicular to the direction of flow to optimize axial resolution, which is typically the parasternal long-axis view for MR jets. VCW of greater than 7 mm is specific for severe MR, whereas VCW of less than 3 mm indicates mild MR.[48] Unfortunately, intermediate values could correspond to MR of any severity, and the grades of severity are separated by small differences in measurement. Unlike the jet area method, VCW does not necessarily underestimate eccentric MR jets.[57] However, the effective regurgitant orifice (ERO) may not be circular but rather crescentic or elliptical, particularly in FMR. The VCW of a noncircular ERO varies depending on imaging plane and may inaccurately grade the severity of MR. In the presence of multiple regurgitant jets, overall MR severity is difficult to assess by the VCW method. Given its static measurement from a single frame, VCW may overestimate severity of late-systolic MR from prolapse.

Proximal Flow Convergence

As blood flow converges proximally to a circular regurgitant orifice, concentric hemispheric shells of increasing velocity and decreasing surface area are formed. Using color Doppler, a hemispheric zone of proximal flow convergence can be outlined by the aliasing threshold, which can be set by shifting the baseline of the color scale or adjusting the Nyquist limit. At this zone of convergence, flow rate is calculated by multiplying the aliasing velocity by the surface area of the hemisphere (proximal isovelocity surface area, or PISA), the radius of which can be measured. Using the continuity equation, the EROA can be calculated by dividing the flow rate by the peak MR velocity, obtained from the CW Doppler tracing (**Fig. 8**). The product

of the EROA and the velocity-time integral (VTI) of the MR jet yields the RVol. An EROA ≥ 0.4 cm^2 and RVol ≥ 60 mL are consistent with severe MR, whereas EROA less than 0.2 cm^2 and RVol less than 30 mL suggest mild MR.[48]

Quantification of MR by the 2D PISA method has several limitations, one of which is the geometric assumption of a circular regurgitant orifice producing hemispheric PISA shells. FMR is associated with a crescentic ERO, typically more elongated along the line of coaptation, resulting in underestimation of severity by 2D PISA.[58,59] PISA hemisphericity is dependent on not only the shape of the ERO but also the distance from the regurgitant orifice (ie, PISA radius) and the planarity of its base. Flows farther from the orifice (aliasing at a low Nyquist limit) converge into an elongated PISA, whereas flows closer to the orifice (aliasing at a high Nyquist limit) converge into a flattened PISA. The base of the PISA hemisphere is typically formed by the relatively flat (180°) valve plane. However, in eccentric jets (eg, due to a flail leaflet), the PISA is prone to overestimation secondary to LA wall constraint, if an angle correction for the conical base of the incomplete PISA hemisphere is not performed.

These geometric assumptions can be obviated by using 3D techniques. Multiplanar reconstructions of 3D color Doppler volumes allow for direct planimetry of the vena contracta area (VCA), which is equivalent to the EROA (**Fig. 9**). Although guidelines on the use of 3D VCA have not yet been established, a threshold of ≥ 0.4 cm^2 has been shown to be highly accurate for identifying severe MR, independent of the cause.[51] Multiple regurgitant jets can be quantified by the cumulative VCA (**Fig. 10**). Alternatively, a nonhemispherical PISA can be contoured from a 3D volume, using specialized software, in order to calculate the EROA.[50] Both the 3D VCA and 3D PISA methods are limited by technical factors, such as susceptibility to color Doppler blooming effect and the reduced spatial and temporal resolution of 3DE.

As with the jet area or VCW method, PISA (2D or 3D) assessment is based on a single systolic frame and does not account for dynamic changes in regurgitant flow and EROA. Variation in the PISA radius throughout systole may result in a wide range of calculated values for EROA and RVol. In order to calculate an accurate maximal EROA, measurement of the PISA radius should be performed at the same time in the cardiac cycle as the peak MR velocity. Non-holosystolic MR (eg, late-systolic MR in prolapse) and temporal variation in regurgitant flow (eg,

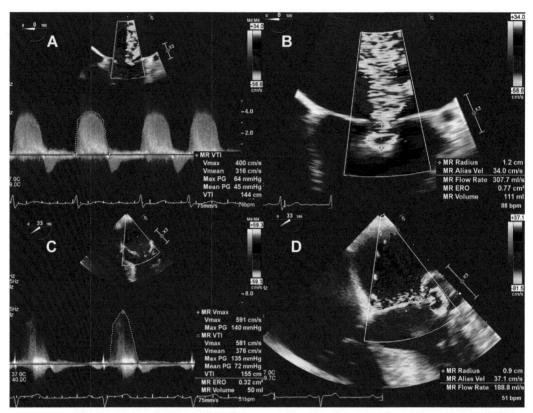

Fig. 8. Quantification of MR with PISA. (*A, B*) FMR with central jet that is amenable to PISA quantification, which calculates EROA of 0.77 cm² and RVol of 111 mL, consistent with severe MR. (*C, D*) Flail leaflet with eccentric MR jet, complicating PISA quantification, due to LA wall constraint. CW Doppler signal suggests non-holosystolic MR, although the beam of interrogation is not well aligned with the jet.

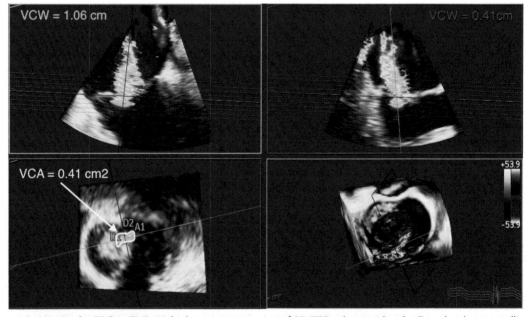

Fig. 9. Noncircular ERO in FMR. Multiplanar reconstruction of 3D TEE volume with color Doppler shows an elliptical ERO, typical of FMR. VCW in one view (*green plane, top left*) measures 1.06 cm, whereas VCW in another (*red plane, top right*) measures 0.41 cm. Planimetry of the cross-sectional area yields a 3D VCA of 0.41 cm², consistent with severe MR.

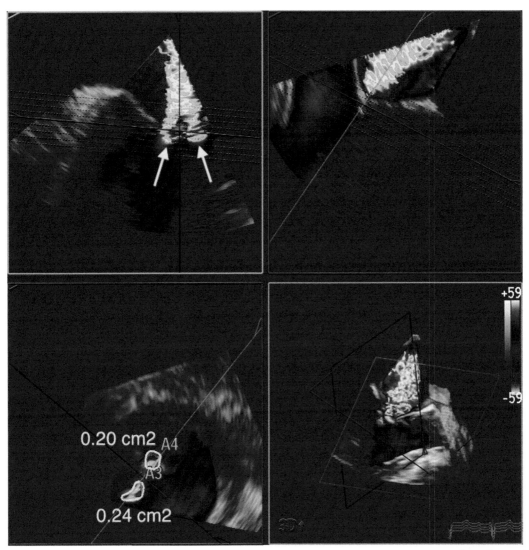

Fig. 10. Multiple regurgitant jets. Quantification of MR with 2 separate jets (*arrows*), using planimetry of VCA from multiplanar reconstruction of 3D TEE color Doppler volume, shows cumulative VCA of 0.20 cm^2 + 0.24 cm^2 = 0.44 cm^2 consistent with severe MR.

bimodal pattern in FMR) impose further challenges to quantification by PISA. In these situations, the maximal instantaneous EROA is not necessarily reflective of MR severity. Instead, the maximal EROA should be normalized to the proportion of systole during which MR occurs, or RVol (which accounts for MR duration in the VTI component) should be used for quantification. Despite these limitations, MR quantification by the PISA method is still less susceptible to changes in instrument settings than other color Doppler methods.[60]

Volumetric Methods

Mitral RVol can also be derived from the difference between the LV total stroke volume (mitral inflow volume) and the forward stroke volume (aortic outflow volume), assuming the absence of significant aortic regurgitation. Mitral inflow volume can be calculated by multiplying the cross-sectional mitral annular area and the mitral inflow VTI. Similarly, the aortic outflow volume is the product of the cross-sectional area and the VTI of the LV outflow tract. Cross-sectional areas of both the mitral annulus and the LV outflow tract are calculated from linear diameter measurements and the assumption of circular geometry, which may lead to inaccuracies. Alternatively, the LV total stroke volume may be derived from LV end-diastolic and end-systolic volumes. Compared with 2D methods, quantitation of LV volumes by 3DE avoids geometric assumptions and underestimation due to apical foreshortening.[61] In the setting of aortic regurgitation, pulmonic outflow volume may be substituted for the forward stroke volume, assuming the lack of significant pulmonic regurgitation. Importantly, the volumetric method quantifies a cumulative RVol, irrespective of the number of regurgitant jets, and is useful for assessing eccentric and non-holosystolic jets that are difficult to quantify by PISA. However, in cases of low stroke volume or small LV chamber, regurgitant fraction (RF) may be a more appropriate metric of MR severity than the RVol. Severe MR corresponds to RF $\geq$50%, whereas mild MR typically has RF less than 30%.[26]

Hemodynamic Signs of Severe Mitral Regurgitation

In a comprehensive evaluation of MR severity, secondary hemodynamic signs of chronic severe MR should be sought and taken into consideration with the quantitative parameters (Table 3). In the setting of primary MR, LA and LV dilatations, as well as pulmonary hypertension, suggest chronic severe MR, although these may be nonspecific. In FMR, these signs of cardiac remodeling may be causative and do not necessarily indicate severe MR. Systolic flow reversal in the pulmonary veins is specific for severe MR (Fig. 11A).[62] However, blunted systolic flow may be due to significant MR, elevated LA pressure from other causes (especially in FMR), decreased LA compliance, or atrial fibrillation. In severe MR, the additional RVol increases mitral inflow, such that the early diastolic velocity (E wave) can exceed 1.2 m/s (Fig. 11B). The E-wave velocity is, however, also influenced by LV diastolic function, LA compliance, and the presence of mitral stenosis. Nonetheless, mitral inflow pattern of a low E-wave velocity with A-wave predominance essentially excludes severe MR.[48]

Cardiac Magnetic Resonance

Further testing is warranted when the severity of MR is uncertain, whether due to discordant parameters or discrepancy between the echocardiographic and clinical findings. Although right heart catheterization may be indicated in this situation, noninvasive quantification of MR can be accomplished with CMR. Qualitatively, a signal void due to spin dephasing proximal to the mitral valve plane on cine long-axis images indicates the presence of MR (Fig. 12A). Quantitation by CMR relies upon an indirect volumetric approach, similar to echocardiography, to calculate mitral RVol and fraction. Subtraction of the aortic outflow volume (obtained by through-plane velocity-encoded imaging) from the total LV stroke volume (derived from planimetry of the short-axis cine images) yields mitral RVol (Fig. 12B–D). In the absence of velocity-encoded sequences, RVol can also be calculated as the difference between the left and right ventricular stroke volumes (from cine imaging). MR quantitation by CMR has not been well validated with clinical outcomes, so the RVol and RF thresholds for regurgitant severity by echocardiography have been adopted for CMR.[52]

In general, CMR has modest correlation with echocardiography for grading MR severity.[63–65] Although RVol tends to be overestimated by PISA as compared with CMR,[63] no such trend exists between CMR and the volumetric method by pulsed-wave Doppler.[64] More discrepancy between the modalities has been noted with grading FMR. Although CMR has higher reproducibility than echocardiography for MR quantification,[63–65] CMR is limited by its higher cost, reduced accessibility (particularly in patients with metallic implants), and inaccuracies in the setting of arrhythmia. In addition, echocardiography allows for assessment of the

Table 3
Quantitative and semiquantitative mitral regurgitation parameters

	Mild MR	Severe MR
Distal jet area	<20%	$\geq$40%
CW Doppler signal	Faint, nonholosystolic	Dense (similar to antegrade), holosystolic
Vena contracta width	<3 mm	$\geq$7 mm
EROA	<0.2 cm^2	$\geq$0.4 cm^2
Regurgitant volume	<30 mL	$\geq$60 mL
Regurgitant fraction	<30%	$\geq$50%
Pulmonary vein flow	Systolic > diastolic wave	Systolic reversal
Mitral inflow	E > A wave	E >1.2 m/s

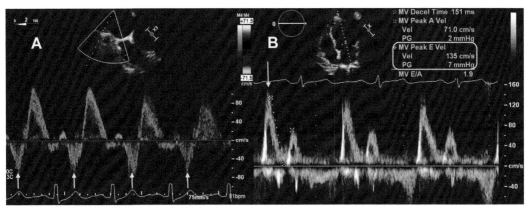

Fig. 11. Secondary signs of severe MR. (*A*) Systolic reversal (*arrows*) of pulmonary vein flow on PW Doppler by TEE. (*B*) Elevated E wave >1.2 cm/s (*arrow*) on PW Doppler of mitral inflow by TTE, in the absence of mitral stenosis, suggesting severe MR. PW, pulsed-wave.

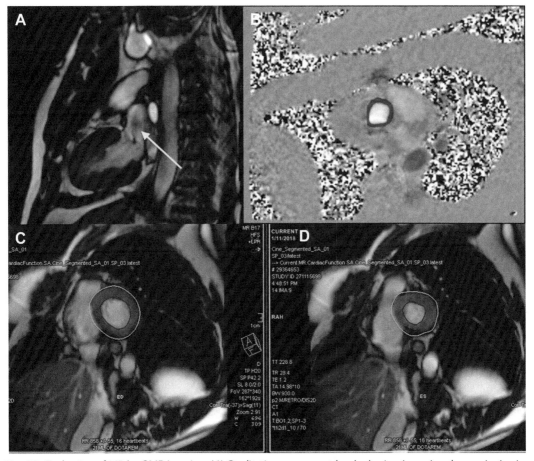

Fig. 12. Evaluation of MR by CMR imaging. (*A*) Qualitative assessment by dephasing (*arrow*) on long-axis cine images. (*B*) Velocity-encoded phase contrast image at the aortic valve plane with region of interest (*red outline*) to determine aortic outflow volume. (*C, D*) Endocardial contouring (*red outline*) of LV cavity on series of short-axis cine images at end-diastole (*C*) and end-systole (*D*) to calculate LVEDV and LVESV. Total LV stroke volume = LVEDV – LVESV. Mitral RVol = Total LV stroke volume – Aortic outflow volume. LVEDV, left ventricular end-diastolic volume; LVESV, left ventricular end-systolic volume.

dynamic physiology of MR and its hemodynamic consequences with exercise stress testing, which can be helpful in gauging the severity of MR.[26]

SUMMARY

MR either results from valvular degeneration or is secondary to myocardial dysfunction. Transcatheter mitral valve repair techniques, especially edge-to-edge leaflet repair, are emerging as feasible therapies for patients with severe MR who are at high risk for surgery. Patient selection is a complex decision requiring a multidisciplinary heart team and depends on clinical factors, anatomic feasibility of repair, and the severity of MR. Echocardiography is the primary diagnostic tool for identification and characterization of both degenerative and FMR mechanisms and for anatomic suitability for transcatheter repair. Quantitation of MR involves integration of multiple echocardiographic parameters and may be further clarified with CMR imaging. Comprehensive evaluation of mitral valve structure and function with imaging may help optimize patient selection for transcatheter mitral valve repair and subsequent clinical outcomes.

SUPPLEMENTARY DATA

Videos related to this article can be found online at https://doi.org/10.1016/j.iccl.2018.04.002.

REFERENCES

1. Nkomo VT, Gardin JM, Skelton TN, et al. Burden of valvular heart diseases: a population-based study. Lancet 2006;368(9540):1005–11.
2. Ling LH, Enriquez-Sarano M, Seward JB, et al. Clinical outcome of mitral regurgitation due to flail leaflet. N Engl J Med 1996;335(19):1417–23.
3. Nishimura RA, McGoon MD, Shub C, et al. Echocardiographically documented mitral-valve prolapse. Long-term follow-up of 237 patients. N Engl J Med 1985;313(21):1305–9.
4. Trichon BH, Felker GM, Shaw LK, et al. Relation of frequency and severity of mitral regurgitation to survival among patients with left ventricular systolic dysfunction and heart failure. Am J Cardiol 2003; 91(5):538–43.
5. Rossi A, Dini FL, Faggiano P, et al. Independent prognostic value of functional mitral regurgitation in patients with heart failure. A quantitative analysis of 1256 patients with ischaemic and non-ischaemic dilated cardiomyopathy. Heart 2011; 97(20):1675–80.
6. Grigioni F, Tribouilloy C, Avierinos JF, et al. Outcomes in mitral regurgitation due to flail leaflets a

multicenter European study. JACC Cardiovasc Imaging 2008;1(2):133–41.
7. Grigioni F, Enriquez-Sarano M, Ling LH, et al. Sudden death in mitral regurgitation due to flail leaflet. J Am Coll Cardiol 1999;34(7):2078–85.
8. Levine RA, Schwammenthal E. Ischemic mitral regurgitation on the threshold of a solution: from paradoxes to unifying concepts. Circulation 2005; 112(5):745–58.
9. Watanabe N, Ogasawara Y, Yamaura Y, et al. Mitral annulus flattens in ischemic mitral regurgitation: geometric differences between inferior and anterior myocardial infarction: a real-time 3-dimensional echocardiographic study. Circulation 2005;112(9 Suppl):I458–62.
10. Otsuji Y, Levine RA, Takeuchi M, et al. Mechanism of ischemic mitral regurgitation. J Cardiol 2008; 51(3):145–56.
11. Gertz ZM, Raina A, Saghy L, et al. Evidence of atrial functional mitral regurgitation due to atrial fibrillation: reversal with arrhythmia control. J Am Coll Cardiol 2011;58(14):1474–81.
12. Carpentier A. Cardiac valve surgery–the "French correction". J Thorac Cardiovasc Surg 1983;86(3): 323–37.
13. Alfieri O, Maisano F, De Bonis M, et al. The double-orifice technique in mitral valve repair: a simple solution for complex problems. J Thorac Cardiovasc Surg 2001;122(4):674–81.
14. Feldman T, Foster E, Glower DD, et al. Percutaneous repair or surgery for mitral regurgitation. N Engl J Med 2011;364(15):1395–406.
15. Feldman T, Kar S, Elmariah S, et al. Randomized comparison of percutaneous repair and surgery for mitral regurgitation: 5-year results of EVEREST II. J Am Coll Cardiol 2015;66(25): 2844–54.
16. Whitlow PL, Feldman T, Pedersen WR, et al. Acute and 12-month results with catheter-based mitral valve leaflet repair: the EVEREST II (endovascular valve edge-to-edge repair) high risk study. J Am Coll Cardiol 2012;59(2):130–9.
17. Lim DS, Reynolds MR, Feldman T, et al. Improved functional status and quality of life in prohibitive surgical risk patients with degenerative mitral regurgitation after transcatheter mitral valve repair. J Am Coll Cardiol 2014;64(2):182–92.
18. Nickenig G, Hammerstingl C, Schueler R, et al. Transcatheter mitral annuloplasty in chronic functional mitral regurgitation: 6-month results with the Cardioband Percutaneous Mitral Repair System. JACC Cardiovasc Interv 2016;9(19): 2039–47.
19. Nickenig G, Schueler R, Dager A, et al. Treatment of chronic functional mitral valve regurgitation with a percutaneous annuloplasty system. J Am Coll Cardiol 2016;67(25):2927–36.

20. Lipiecki J, Siminiak T, Sievert H, et al. Coronary sinus-based percutaneous annuloplasty as treatment for functional mitral regurgitation: the TITAN II trial. Open Heart 2016;3(2):e000411.

21. Seeburger J, Rinaldi M, Nielsen SL, et al. Off-pump transapical implantation of artificial neochordae to correct mitral regurgitation: the TACT Trial (Transapical Artificial Chordae Tendinae) proof of concept. J Am Coll Cardiol 2014; 63(9):914–9.

22. Gammie JS, Wilson P, Bartus K, et al. Transapical beating-heart mitral valve repair with an expanded polytetrafluoroethylene cordal implantation device: initial clinical experience. Circulation 2016;134(3): 189–97.

23. Bapat V, Rajagopal V, Meduri C, et al. Early experience with new transcatheter mitral valve replacement. J Am Coll Cardiol 2018;71(1):12–21.

24. Regueiro A, Granada JF, Dagenais F, et al. Transcatheter mitral valve replacement: insights from early clinical experience and future challenges. J Am Coll Cardiol 2017;69(17):2175–92.

25. Nishimura RA, Otto CM, Bonow RO, et al. 2014 AHA/ACC guideline for the management of patients with valvular heart disease: a report of the American College of Cardiology/American Heart Association Task Force on practice guidelines. Circulation 2014;129(23):e521–643.

26. O'Gara PT, Grayburn PA, Badhwar V, et al. 2017 ACC expert consensus decision pathway on the management of mitral regurgitation: a report of the American College of Cardiology Task Force on expert consensus decision pathways. J Am Coll Cardiol 2017;70(19):2421–49.

27. Stone GW, Vahanian AS, Adams DH, et al. Clinical trial design principles and endpoint definitions for transcatheter mitral valve repair and replacement: part 1: clinical trial design principles: a consensus document from the mitral valve academic research consortium. J Am Coll Cardiol 2015;66:278–307.

28. Wu AH, Aaronson KD, Bolling SF, et al. Impact of mitral valve annuloplasty on mortality risk in patients with mitral regurgitation and left ventricular systolic dysfunction. J Am Coll Cardiol 2005;45(3): 381–7.

29. Mihaljevic T, Lam B-K, Rajeswaran J, et al. Impact of mitral valve annuloplasty combined with revascularization in patients with functional ischemic mitral regurgitation. J Am Coll Cardiol 2007; 49(22):2191–201.

30. Hahn RT, Abraham T, Adams MS, et al. Guidelines for performing a comprehensive transesophageal echocardiographic examination: recommendations from the American Society of Echocardiography and the Society of Cardiovascular Anesthesiologists. J Am Soc Echocardiogr 2013;26:921–64.

31. Carpentier AF, Pellerin M, Fuzellier JF, et al. Extensive calcification of the mitral valve anulus: pathology and surgical management. J Thorac Cardiovasc Surg 1996;111(4):718–29 [discussion: 729–30].

32. Grewal J, Suri R, Mankad S, et al. Mitral annular dynamics in myxomatous valve disease: new insights with real-time 3-dimensional echocardiography. Circulation 2010;121(12):1423–31.

33. Chandra S, Salgo IS, Sugeng L, et al. Characterization of degenerative mitral valve disease using morphologic analysis of real-time three-dimensional echocardiographic images: objective insight into complexity and planning of mitral valve repair. Circ Cardiovasc Imaging 2011;4(1):24–32.

34. Watanabe N, Ogasawara Y, Yamaura Y, et al. Quantitation of mitral valve tenting in ischemic mitral regurgitation by transthoracic real-time three-dimensional echocardiography. J Am Coll Cardiol 2005;45(5):763–9.

35. Golba K, Mokrzycki K, Drozdz J, et al. Mechanisms of functional mitral regurgitation in ischemic cardiomyopathy determined by transesophageal echocardiography (from the surgical treatment for Ischemic Heart Failure Trial). Am J Cardiol 2013; 112(11):1812–8.

36. Ahmad RM, Gillinov AM, McCarthy PM, et al. Annular geometry and motion in human ischemic mitral regurgitation: novel assessment with three-dimensional echocardiography and computer reconstruction. Ann Thorac Surg 2004;78(6):2063–8 [discussion: 2068].

37. Kwan J, Shiota T, Agler DA, et al. Geometric differences of the mitral apparatus between ischemic and dilated cardiomyopathy with significant mitral regurgitation: real-time three-dimensional echocardiography study. Circulation 2003;107(8):1135–40.

38. Hung J, Otsuji Y, Handschumacher MD, et al. Mechanism of dynamic regurgitant orifice area variation in functional mitral regurgitation: physiologic insights from the proximal flow convergence technique. J Am Coll Cardiol 1999;33(2):538–45.

39. Herrmann HC, Kar S, Siegel R, et al. Effect of percutaneous mitral repair with the MitraClip device on mitral valve area and gradient. EuroIntervention 2009;4(4):437–42.

40. Mauri L, Garg P, Massaro JM, et al. The EVEREST II Trial: design and rationale for a randomized study of the evalve mitraclip system compared with mitral valve surgery for mitral regurgitation. Am Heart J 2010;160(1):23–9.

41. Cavalcante JL, Rodriguez LL, Kapadia S, et al. Role of echocardiography in percutaneous mitral valve interventions. JACC Cardiovasc Imaging 2012;5(7): 733–46.

42. Perpetua EM, Levin DB, Reisman M. Anatomy and function of the normal and diseased mitral

apparatus: implications for transcatheter therapy. Interv Cardiol Clin 2016;5(1):1–16.

43. Attizzani GF, Ohno Y, Capodanno D, et al. Extended use of percutaneous edge-to-edge mitral valve repair beyond EVEREST (Endovascular Valve Edge-to-Edge Repair) criteria: 30-day and 12-month clinical and echocardiographic outcomes from the GRASP (Getting Reduction of Mitral Insufficiency by Percutaneous Clip Implantation) registry. JACC Cardiovasc Interv 2015;8(1 Pt A):74–82.

44. Estévez-Loureiro R, Franzen O, Winter R, et al. Echocardiographic and clinical outcomes of central versus noncentral percutaneous edge-to-edge repair of degenerative mitral regurgitation. J Am Coll Cardiol 2013;62(25):2370–7.

45. Hanson ID, Hanzel GS, Shannon FL. Mitral valve repair after annuloplasty ring dehiscence using MitraClip. Catheter Cardiovasc Interv 2016;88(2):301–6.

46. Fuchs FC, Hammerstingl C, Werner N, et al. Catheter-based edge-to-edge mitral valve repair after partial rupture of surgical annuloplasty ring. JACC Cardiovasc Interv 2015;8(15):e263–4.

47. Hahn RT. Transcathether valve replacement and valve repair: review of procedures and intraprocedural echocardiographic imaging. Circ Res 2016; 119(2):341–56.

48. Zoghbi WA, Adams D, Bonow RO, et al. Recommendations for noninvasive evaluation of native valvular regurgitation: a report from the American Society of Echocardiography developed in collaboration with the Society for Cardiovascular Magnetic Resonance. J Am Soc Echocardiogr 2017;30(4): 303–71.

49. Little SH. The vena contracta area: conquering quantification with a 3D cut? JACC Cardiovasc Imaging 2012;5(7):677–80.

50. Little SH, Igo SR, Pirat B, et al. In vitro validation of real-time three-dimensional color Doppler echocardiography for direct measurement of proximal isovelocity surface area in mitral regurgitation. Am J Cardiol 2007;99(10):1440–7.

51. Zeng X, Levine RA, Hua L, et al. Diagnostic value of vena contracta area in the quantification of mitral regurgitation severity by color Doppler 3D echocardiography. Circ Cardiovasc Imaging 2011;4(5):506–13.

52. Zoghbi WA, Enriquez-Sarano M, Foster E, et al. Recommendations for evaluation of the severity of native valvular regurgitation with two-dimensional and Doppler echocardiography. J Am Soc Echocardiogr 2003;16(7):777–802.

53. Enriquez-Sarano M, Tajik AJ, Bailey KR, et al. Color flow imaging compared with quantitative Doppler assessment of severity of mitral regurgitation: influence of eccentricity of jet and mechanism of regurgitation. J Am Coll Cardiol 1993;21(5):1211–9.

54. Chen CG, Thomas JD, Anconina J, et al. Impact of impinging wall jet on color Doppler quantification

of mitral regurgitation. Circulation 1991;84(2): 712–20.

55. Utsunomiya T, Patel D, Doshi R, et al. Can signal intensity of the continuous wave Doppler regurgitant jet estimate severity of mitral regurgitation? Am Heart J 1992;123(1):166–71.

56. Topilsky Y, Michelena H, Bichara V, et al. Mitral valve prolapse with mid-late systolic mitral regurgitation: pitfalls of evaluation and clinical outcome compared with holosystolic regurgitation. Circulation 2012;125(13):1643–51.

57. Hall SA, Brickner ME, Willett DL, et al. Assessment of mitral regurgitation severity by Doppler color flow mapping of the vena contracta. Circulation 1997;95(3):636–42.

58. Chandra S, Salgo IS, Sugeng L, et al. A three-dimensional insight into the complexity of flow convergence in mitral regurgitation: adjunctive benefit of anatomic regurgitant orifice area. Am J Physiol Heart Circ Physiol 2011;301(3):H1015–24.

59. Kahlert P, Plicht B, Schenk IM, et al. Direct assessment of size and shape of noncircular vena contracta area in functional versus organic mitral regurgitation using real-time three-dimensional echocardiography. J Am Soc Echocardiogr 2008;21(8):912–21.

60. Utsunomiya T, Ogawa T, Doshi R, et al. Doppler color flow "proximal isovelocity surface area" method for estimating volume flow rate: effects of orifice shape and machine factors. J Am Coll Cardiol 1991;17(5):1103–11.

61. Lang RM, Badano LP, Mor-Avi V, et al. Recommendations for cardiac chamber quantification by echocardiography in adults: an update from the American Society of Echocardiography and the European Association of Cardiovascular Imaging. J Am Soc Echocardiogr 2015;28(1):1–39.e14.

62. Enriquez-Sarano M, Dujardin KS, Tribouilloy CM, et al. Determinants of pulmonary venous flow reversal in mitral regurgitation and its usefulness in determining the severity of regurgitation. Am J Cardiol 1999;83(4):535–41.

63. Uretsky S, Gillam L, Lang R, et al. Discordance between echocardiography and MRI in the assessment of mitral regurgitation severity: a prospective multicenter trial. J Am Coll Cardiol 2015;65(11):1078–88.

64. Lopez-Mattei JC, Ibrahim H, Shaikh KA, et al. Comparative assessment of mitral regurgitation severity by transthoracic echocardiography and cardiac magnetic resonance using an integrative and quantitative approach. Am J Cardiol 2016; 117(2):264–70.

65. Cawley PJ, Hamilton-Craig C, Owens DS, et al. Prospective comparison of valve regurgitation quantitation by cardiac magnetic resonance imaging and transthoracic echocardiography. Circ Cardiovasc Imaging 2013;6(1):48–57.

Percutaneous Balloon Mitral Valvuloplasty
Echocardiographic Eligibility and Procedural Guidance

Jonathan J. Passeri, MD*, Jacob P. Dal-Bianco, MD

KEYWORDS

- Mitral valve • Mitral stenosis • Valvuloplasty • Rheumatic heart disease • Echocardiography

KEY POINTS

- Rheumatic mitral stenosis is a common disease in the developing world and is a significant cause of cardiovascular death or disability.
- Percutaneous balloon mitral valvuloplasty (PBMV) is an effective treatment for rheumatic mitral stenosis.
- Echocardiography plays an important role in the diagnosis of rheumatic mitral stenosis, determining eligibility, guiding, and assessing the outcome of PBMV.

INTRODUCTION

Rheumatic heart disease remains a common and preventable cause of cardiovascular death and morbidity worldwide, particularly in developing countries.[1–3] Rheumatic fever is a late sequela of group A β-hemolytic streptococcal infection. Streptococcal antigen is similar to a glycoprotein found in valve and endocardial tissue. In susceptible hosts, autoantibodies are formed following streptococcal infection that can lead to an inflammatory process known as acute rheumatic fever. Rheumatic carditis occurs in 60% to 90% of cases of acute rheumatic fever, and rheumatic heart disease is a chronic manifestation of rheumatic carditis.[4] Although all of the cardiac valves may be involved in rheumatic heart disease, the mitral valve is most commonly and severely affected, and rheumatic heart disease remains the most common cause of mitral stenosis. The inflammatory process affecting the mitral valve leads to progressive fibrosis of the leaflet, subvalvular chords and leaflet coaptation zones, leading to chordal shortening, fusion of the commissures, and ultimately narrowing of the mitral orifice at the leaflet tips. The stenotic mitral orifice results in increased resistance to transmitral flow. Uncorrected progressive mitral stenosis can eventually lead to disabling symptoms (eg, dyspnea or hemoptysis), pulmonary edema, pulmonary hypertension, right-sided heart failure, atrial fibrillation, thromboembolism, and cardiovascular death.[5,6]

Historically, most patients with symptomatic mitral stenosis were treated with surgical mitral commissurotomy or mitral valve replacement. In 1984, a Japanese cardiac surgeon named Kanji Inuoe first described the technique of balloon mitral valvuloplasty.[7] The technique for performing the procedure was refined in the years that followed. Percutaneous balloon mitral valvuloplasty (PBMV) has since proven to be an effective treatment for rheumatic mitral stenosis, resulting in

Disclosure Statement: None.

Heart Valve Program, Corrigan Minehan Heart Center, Massachusetts General Hospital, Yawkey Building Suite 5B, 55 Fruit Street, Boston, MA 02114, USA

* Corresponding author. Massachusetts General Hospital, Yawkey Building Suite 5700, 55 Fruit Street, Boston, MA 02114.

E-mail address: jpasseri@mgh.harvard.edu

hemodynamic and clinical improvement.[8–11] PBMV has demonstrated equivalent results and restenosis rates compared with surgical mitral commissurotomy.[12,13] Echocardiography plays an important role in all aspects of PBMV, from the initial diagnosis of rheumatic mitral stenosis to determination of suitability for PBMV, guidance of PBMV, and postprocedural assessment.

ECHOCARDIOGRAPHIC FEATURES OF RHEUMATIC MITRAL STENOSIS

The characteristic imaging features of chronic rheumatic mitral stenosis include: (1) doming of the anterior mitral leaflet, where the narrowest orifice is at the leaflet tips creating a hockey stick deformity of the anterior mitral leaflet, (2) restricted mobility or immobility of the posterior mitral leaflets, (3) a fish mouth opening appearance of the mitral valve orifice caused by fusion of the commissures, and (4) subvalvular thickening and chordal shortening (Box 1, Figs. 1 and 2). Doppler echocardiography is used to estimate the transmitral valve gradients (Fig. 3). The mitral valve area can be calculated using the pressure half-time method or measured by direct planimetry of the mitral orifice. Echocardiography is also used to determine the severity of mitral regurgitation.

The outcomes from PBMV are variable and highly dependent on the anatomic characteristics of the valve. When considering intervention for mitral stenosis, one has to carefully evaluate the anatomy of the mitral valve to determine the

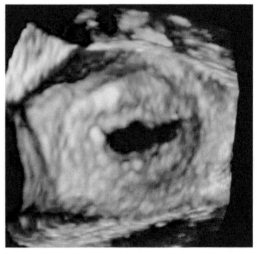

Fig. 2. Three-dimensional transesophageal echocardiographic view of the mitral valve demonstrating the typical fish mouth appearance characteristic of rheumatic mitral stenosis.

Box 1
Characteristic features of rheumatic mitral stenosis

- Hockey stick deformity of the anterior mitral leaflet
- Restricted mobility of the posterior mitral leaflet
- Fish-mouth appearance of the mitral valve orifice
- Subvalvular thickening and chordal shortening

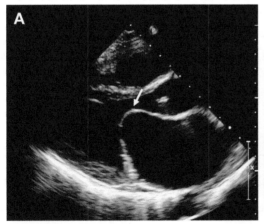
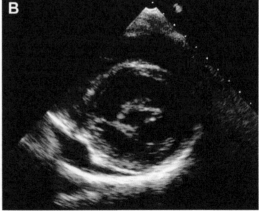

Fig. 1. Echocardiographic features of rheumatic mitral stenosis. (A) the arrow points to doming of the anterior mitral valve leaflet, resulting in a characteristic hockey stick deformity of the anterior leaflet. (B) Fish mouth appearance of the mitral orifice due to fusion of the commissures.

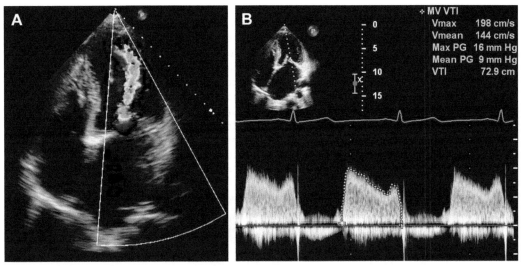

Fig. 3. Transthoracic echocardiogram demonstrating rheumatic mitral stenosis. (A) Color Doppler during mid-diastole demonstrates flow acceleration toward the stenotic mitral orifice at the leaflet tips. (B) Transmitral continuous wave Doppler demonstrating elevated gradients across the mitral valve at a relatively low heart rate consistent with severe mitral stenosis.

feasibility and safety of the PBMV. Morphologic features of the mitral valve assessed by echocardiography have been shown to predict the success of PBMV. The first and most widely used echocardiographic scoring system to predict success of PBMV is known as the Wilkins score.[14] In the Wilkins score, 4 morphologic features of the mitral valve apparatus (leaflet mobility, leaflet thickening, leaflet calcification, and subvalvular thickening) are each assigned a score from 1 to 4 for a total maximum possible score of 16 (Table 1). A score of 8 or less is associated with

Table 1
Grading of mitral valve characteristics from the echocardiographic examination according to the Wilkins classification

Grade	Mobility	Subvalvular Thickening	Thickening	Calcification
1	Highly mobile valve with only leaflet tips restricted	Minimal thickening just below the mitral leaflets	Leaflets near normal in thickness (4–5 mm)	A single area of increased echo brightness
2	Leaflet mid and base portions have normal mobility	Thickening of chordal structures extending up to one-third of the chordal length	Midleaflets normal, considerable thickening of margins (5–8 mm)	Scattered areas of brightness confined to leaflet margins
3	Valve continues to move forward in diastole mainly from the base	Thickening extending to the distal third of the chords	Thickening extending through the entire leaflet (5–8 mm)	Brightness extending into the midportion of the leaflets
4	No or minimal forward movement of the leaflets in diastole	Extensive thickening and shortening of all chordal structures extending down to the papillary muscles	Considerable of all leaflet tissue (>8–10 mm)	Extensive brightness throughout much of the leaflet tissue

The total echocardiographic score was derived from an analysis of mitral leaflet mobility, valvular and subvalvular thickening, and calcification, which were graded from 1 to 4 according to the above criteria, giving a total score of up to 16.

Adapted from Wilkins GT, Weyman AE, Abascal VM, et al. Percutaneous balloon dilatation of the mitral valve: an analysis of echocardiographic variables related to outcome and the mechanism of dilatation. Br Heart J 1988;60(4):300; with permission.

favorable PBMV outcomes. Conversely, a score greater than 8 is associated with poor outcomes from PBMV (Fig. 4). The development of severe mitral regurgitation following PBMV is an important cause of death or disability. Significant bilateral or asymmetric calcium patterns in the commissures are associated with the development of significant mitral regurgitation following PBMV (Figs. 5 and 6).[15,16] Padial and colleagues[15] refined the Wilkins score to incorporate the commissural calcium pattern to predict severe mitral regurgitation after PMV (Box 2).

Both the Wilkins and Padial scoring systems rely on the qualitative and semiquantitative assessment of mitral valve morphologic features, which are subject to interobserver variability and are less reliable for predicting success with scores in the mid-range. In vitro studies have demonstrated that the mechanism by which PBMV helps resolve rheumatic mitral stenosis is by splitting the fused commissures.[17] As such, a valve with a greater extent of commissural fusion may benefit more from PBMV than a valve without any

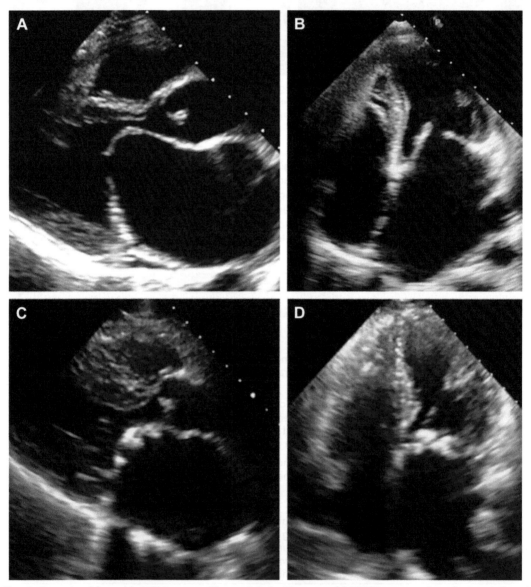

Fig. 4. Example of favorable Wlikins score (5) associated with successful PBMV outcome (panels *A* and *B*) and an unfavorable Wilkins score (13) associated with poor PBMV outcome (panels *C* and *D*). Note the difference in thickening and calcification between these valves. (*Reprinted by permission from* Springer Nature. Hung JW, Park YH. Percutaneous mitral valvulotomy. In: Picard M, Passeri J, Dal-Bianco J, editors. Intraprocedural imaging of cardiovascular interventions; 2016.)

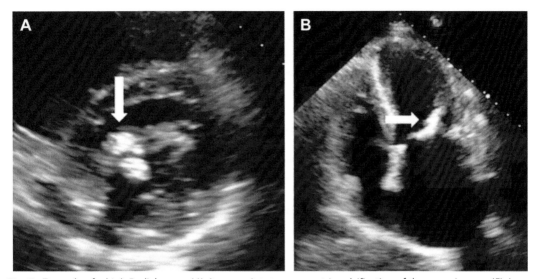

Fig. 5. Example of a high Padial score. (A) Arrow points to asymmetric calcification of the commissures. (B) Arrow points to extensive thickening and shortening of the chordae extending to the papillary muscle. A high Padial score is associated with an increased risk of severe mitral regurgitation. (*Reprinted by permission from* Springer Nature. Hung JW, Park YH. Percutaneous mitral valvulotomy. In: Picard M, Passeri J, Dal-Bianco J, editors. Intraprocedural imaging of cardiovascular interventions; 2016.)

commissural fusion, in which the stenosis is due to rigid leaflets or annular narrowing. In the latter circumstance, the leaflets or subvalvular apparatus may fracture during PBMV, resulting in worsening mitral regurgitation. Nunes and colleagues[18] demonstrated improved accuracy for predicting success with PBMV and the development of worsening mitral regurgitation using the commissural area ratio and leaflet displacement measurement. These quantitative criteria incorporate both functional and morphologic features of rheumatic mitral stenosis to predict PBMV success and the likelihood of causing severe mitral regurgitation. A commissural area ratio of greater than 1.25 and leaflet displacement

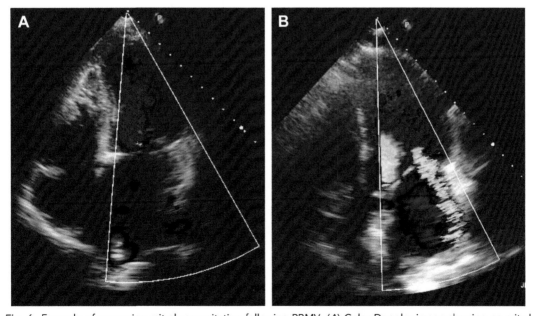

Fig. 6. Example of worsening mitral regurgitation following PBMV. (A) Color Doppler image showing no mitral regurgitation prior to PBMV. (B) Color Doppler image demonstrating significant mitral regurgitation following PBMV.

Box 2
Echocardiogram score for severe mitral regurgitation after percutaneous mitral valvuloplasty according to the Padial method

I-II. Valvular thickening (score each leaflet separately)

  1. Leaflet near normal (4–5 mm) or with only a thick segment

  2. Leaflet fibrotic and/or calcified evenly; no thin areas

  3. Leaflet fibrotic and/or calcified with uneven distribution; thinner segments are mildly thickened (5–8 mm)

  4. Leaflet fibrotic and/or calcified with uneven distribution; thinner segments are near normal (4–5 mm)

III. Commissural calcification

  1. Fibrosis and/or calcium in only 1 commissure

  2. Both commissures mildly affected

  3. Calcium in both commissures, 1 markedly affected

  4. Calcium in both commissures, both markedly affected

IV. Subvalvular disease

  1. Minimal thickening of chordal structures just below the valve

  2. Thickening of chordae extending up to one-third of chordal length

  3. Thickening to the distal third of the chordae

  4. Extensive thickening and shortening of all chordae extending down to the papillary muscle

The total score is the sum of these echocardiographic features (maximum 16).
Adapted from Padial LR, Freitas N, Sagie A, et al. Echocardiography can predict which patients will develop severe mitral regurgitation after percutaneous mitral valvulotomy. J Am Coll Cardiol 1996;27(5):1226; with permission.

---

of less than or equal to 12 mm are associated with poor outcomes from PBMV. An important limitation to all of these scoring systems is that none of them incorporates the severity of mitral regurgitation at baseline. Moderate or severe mitral regurgitation at baseline is a considered a contraindication to PMBV.

INTRAPROCEDURAL GUIDANCE FOR PECUTANEOUS BALLOON MITRAL VALVULOPLASTY

Prior to PBMV, a complete transthoracic echocardiogram should be obtained to evaluate suitability for the procedure. A transesophageal echocardiogram (TEE) is typically performed immediately prior to PBMV to exclude thrombus within the left atrium or left atrial appendage. Patients with left atrial or left atrial appendage thrombus should not undergo PBMV except in special circumstances (Fig. 7). TEE or intracardiac echocardiography (ICE) can be useful for guiding the transseptal puncture, particularly in patients with severely dilated atria or abnormal interatrial septum anatomy. The optimal location for transseptal puncture for PBMV is in the middle or slightly posterior aspect of the fossa ovalis. TEE or ICE can also visualize the transseptal needle and/or catheter within the left atrium and confirm successful puncture of the interatrial septum (Fig. 8).

A critical factor in performing PBMV is selecting the appropriate balloon size. An undersized balloon may not alleviate the stenosis, whereas an oversized balloon may cause excessive damage to the commissures, leaflets, or subvalvular

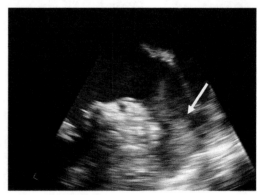

Fig. 7. Transesophageal echocardiogram demonstrating a thrombus within the left atrial appendage (*white arrow*).

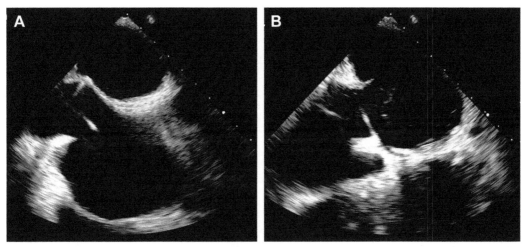

Fig. 8. Transesophageal echocardiogram to guide the transseptal puncture. (A) The location of the transseptal need prior to puncture is noted by indentation of the interatrial septum. The location of the needle is in the middle of the fossa ovalis. (B) Transseptal needle noted in the left atrium, confirming successful puncture of the interatrial septum.

apparatus, leading to severe mitral regurgitation. Using patient height or body surface area are common methods for selecting balloon size. However, the relationship between height and diameter of the mitral orifice is nonlinear. Some investigators have proposed using the mitral annular diameter measured by echocardiography or distance between the 2 commissures in the apical 2-chamber view to select the optimal balloon size.[19]

Echocardiography is performed during PBMV to help achieve an optimal result and rapidly assess for potential complications. After each successive balloon inflation, echocardiographic images (typically transthoracic) are obtained to determine the transmitral valve gradients and severity of mitral regurgitation. Echocardiography is also used throughout and at the conclusion of the procedure to evaluate for the development of a pericardial effusion, as perforation leading to cardiac tamponade may occur as a complication of PBMV.

POSTPERCUTANEOUS BALLOON MITRAL VALVULOPLASTY IMAGING

Following PBMV, echocardiography should be performed to estimate the transmitral valve gradients, measure the mitral valve area, and determine the severity of mitral regurgitation (Fig. 9). The incidence of severe mitral regurgitation has been reported to be between 1% and 9% following PMV.[20,21] The mechanism of severe mitral regurgitation after PMV is most often due to leaflet tears, and the

postprocedure echocardiogram, like the preprocedural echocardiogram, should carefully assess leaflet mobility and morphology. In the near term following PBMV, the mitral valve area should be measured by direct planimetry rather than calculated by the pressure half-time method. The pressure half-time is highly dependent on chamber compliance, which changes dramatically over time after PBMV. The pressure half-time method for calculating mitral valve area has been shown to be inaccurate immediately after PBMV before chamber compliance has had sufficient time to adjust to relief of stenosis.[22]

SUMMARY

PBMV offers an effective therapy for rheumatic mitral stenosis in selected patients. Echocardiography is not only the primary method used to establish the diagnosis of rheumatic mitral stenosis, but also plays a central role in all aspects of PBMV. The success of PBMV depends on the echocardiographic assessment of the pliability of the leaflets, the degree of degeneration and calcification of the commissures, subvalvular apparatus, annulus, and valve leaflets, and determination of the degree of mitral regurgitation at baseline. During the procedure, echocardiography is used to exclude left atrial thrombus, ensure optimal transseptal puncture, select the appropriate balloon size, determine the change in hemodynamics and degree of mitral regurgitation following each balloon inflation, and rapidly identify complications. Following PMBV,

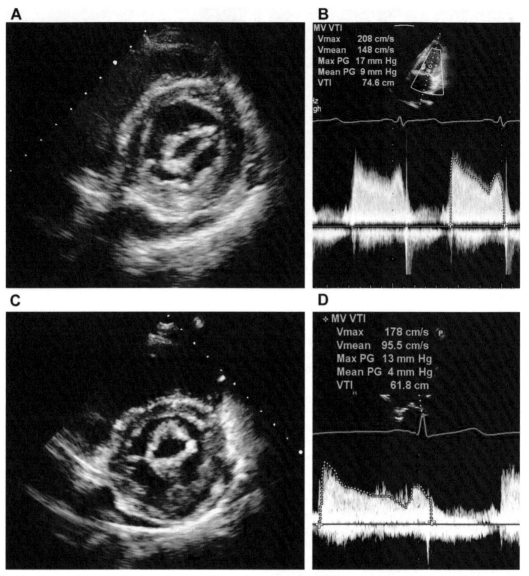

Fig. 9. Echocardiographic images prior to and immediately following PBMV. (*A*) Echocardiographic short axis view of the stenotic mitral orifice and (*B*) transmitral gradients prior to PBMV. Following PBMV, (*C*) the mitral orifice opening has improved, and (*D*) the transmitral gradients are significantly reduced.

echocardiography is used to assess the results and follow patients prospectively.

REFERENCES

1. Iung B, Baron G, Butchart EG, et al. A prospective survey of patients with valvular heart disease in Europe: the Euro Heart Survey on valvular heart disease. Eur Heart J 2003;24(13):1231–43.
2. Roth GA, Johnson C, Abajobir A, et al. Global, regional, and national burden of cardiovascular diseases for 10 causes, 1990 to 2015. J Am Coll Cardiol 2017;70(1):1–25.
3. Carapetis JR, Steer AC, Mulholland EK, et al. The global burden of group A streptococcal diseases. Lancet Infect Dis 2005;5(11):685–94.
4. Carapetis JR, McDonald M, Wilson NJ. Acute rheumatic fever. Lancet 2005;366(9480):155–68.
5. Wilson JK, Greenwood WF. The natural history of mitral stenosis. Can Med Assoc J 1954;71(4):323–31.
6. Rinkevich D, Lessick J, Mutlak D, et al. Natural history of moderate mitral valve stenosis. Isr Med Assoc J 2003;5(1):15–8.
7. Inoue K, Owaki T, Nakamura T, et al. Clinical application of transvenous mitral commissurotomy by a new balloon catheter. J Thorac Cardiovasc Surg 1984;87(3):394–402.

8. Ben Farhat M, Ayari M, Maatouk F, et al. Percutaneous balloon versus surgical closed and open mitral commissurotomy: seven-year follow-up results of a randomized trial. Circulation 1998;97(3):245–50.

9. Iung B, Garbarz E, Michaud P, et al. Late results of percutaneous mitral commissurotomy in a series of 1024 patients. Analysis of late clinical deterioration: frequency, anatomic findings, and predictive factors. Circulation 1999;99(25):3272–8.

10. de Souza JA, Martinez EE Jr, Ambrose JA, et al. Percutaneous balloon mitral valvuloplasty in comparison with open mitral valve commissurotomy for mitral stenosis during pregnancy. J Am Coll Cardiol 2001;37(3):900–3.

11. Iung B, Nicoud-Houel A, Fondard O, et al. Temporal trends in percutaneous mitral commissurotomy over a 15-year period. Eur Heart J 2004;25(8):701–7.

12. Turi ZG, Reyes VP, Raju BS, et al. Percutaneous balloon versus surgical closed commissurotomy for mitral stenosis. A prospective, randomized trial. Circulation 1991;83(4):1179–85.

13. Arora R, Nair M, Kalra GS, et al. Immediate and long-term results of balloon and surgical closed mitral valvotomy: a randomized comparative study. Am Heart J 1993;125(4):1091–4.

14. Wilkins GT, Weyman AE, Abascal VM, et al. Pecutaneous balloon dilatation of the mitral valve: an analysis of echocardiographic variables related to outcorme and the mechanism of dilatation. Br Heart J 1988;60(4):299–308.

15. Padial LR, Freitas N, Sagie A, et al. Echocardiography can predict which patients will develop severe mitral regurgitation after percutaneous mitral valvulotomy. J Am Coll Cardiol 1996; 27(5):1225–31.

16. Cannan CR, Nishimura RA, Reeder GS, et al. Echocardiographic assessment of commissural calcium: a simple predictor of outcome after percutaneous mitral balloon valvotomy. J Am Coll Cardiol 1997; 29(1):175–80.

17. Ribeiro PA, al Zaibag M, Rajendran V, et al. Mechanism of mitral valve area increase by in vitro single and double balloon mitral valvotomy. Am J Cardiol 1988;62(4):264–9.

18. Nunes MC, Tan TC, Elmariah S, et al. The echo score revisited: impact of incorporating commissural morphology and leaflet displacement to the prediction of outcome for patients undergoing percutaneous mitral valvuloplasty. Circulation 2014;129(8):886–95.

19. Sanati HR, Kiavar M, Salehi N, et al. Percutaneous mitral valvuloplasty–a new method for balloon sizing based on maximal commissural diameter to improve procedural results. Am Heart Hosp J 2010;8(1):29–32.

20. Palacios IF, Sanchez PL, Harrell LC, et al. Which patients benefit from percutaneous mitral balloon valvuloplasty? Prevalvuloplasty and postvalvuloplasty variables that predict long-term outcome. Circulation 2002;105(12):1465–71.

21. Chen CR, Cheng TO. Percutaneous balloon mitral valvuloplasty by the Inoue technique: a multicenter study of 4832 patients in China. Am Heart J 1995; 129(6):1197–203.

22. Thomas JD, Wilkins GT, Choong CY, et al. Inaccuracy of mitral pressure half-time immediately after percutaneous mitral valvotomy. Dependence on transmitral gradient and left atrial and ventricular compliance. Circulation 1988; 78(4):980–93.

Three-Dimensional Printing for Planning of Structural Heart Interventions

Dee Dee Wang, MD[a,*], Neil Gheewala, MD[a],
Rajan Shah, MD[a], Dmitry Levin, BS[b], Eric Myers, BFA[a],
Marianne Rollet, BS, RT(R)(CT)[a], William W. O'Neill, MD[a]

KEYWORDS

• CT • 3D printing • Structural heart • Transcatheter

KEY POINTS

- Three-dimensional (3D) printing is a process leading to the creation of a physical 3D model to be used for teaching, patient education, device evaluation, and procedural planning.
- 3D-printed models of patient-specific anatomy can be generated from 3D transesophageal (TEE), cardiac MRI, or cardiac computed tomography (CT) datasets.
- Although TEE and MRI can be used to provide 3D datasets, CT imaging with contrast is preferred because it provides reproducible quality and detailed anatomic information on size and function in an established Digital Imaging and Communications in Medicine (DICOM) format that can be efficiently converted to a printable file.
- Through a process termed segmentation, dedicated medical software creates a final surface model from the original DICOM file into a final stereolithographic dataset.
- 3D printing can be applied to a range of structural heart procedures to enhance patient screening and to identify an optimal procedural approach, including perivalvular leak closure, percutaneous left atrial appendage occlusion, and transcatheter mitral valve replacement.

INTRODUCTION

Three-dimensional (3D) printing has long been associated with the manufacturing of custom implants, product lines, and surgical guides.[1] In medicine, 3D printing in structural heart interventions is relatively new and fills an imaging void created by transcatheter therapies.

With the increase in structural heart interventions, imaging has lagged behind in the understanding of human anatomy. In traditional open-heart surgery, surgeons do not depend on imaging for guidance of suture placement or valve implantation. Surgeons can cut open the chest cavity and palpate all the cardiac structures and valvular defects. In transcatheter therapies, patients are typically not candidates for traditional open-heart surgery owing to frailty and hence are referred for transluminal options.[2] This takes the physicians' ability to palpate anatomy away from the operating room. Hence, imaging the anatomy of interest is crucial to therapy success. However, imaging alone does not solve the understanding of

Disclosures: Dr D.D. Wang is a consultant for Edwards LifeSciences, Boston Scientific, and Materialise. Dr D.D. Wang also provides computed tomography (CT) core laboratory services through Henry Ford Hospital to the MITRAL trial, and CT and Echo core laboratory services through Henry Ford Hospital to the NIH sponsored LAMPOON clinical trial. Dr W.W. O'Neill has received research support from Edwards Lifesciences. Dr W.W. O'Neill is a consultant for Edwards Lifesciences. All other authors report no relevant financial disclosures.
[a] Center for Structural Heart Disease, Henry Ford Hospital, 2799 West Grand Boulevard, Clara Ford Pavilion, 4th Floor, 432, Detroit, MI 48202, USA; [b] Department of Medicine, Section of Cardiology, University of Washington Medical Center, 1959 Northeast Pacific Street, Box 356422, Seattle, WA 98195, USA
* Corresponding author.
E-mail address: dwang2@hfhs.org

Intervent Cardiol Clin 7 (2018) 415–423
https://doi.org/10.1016/j.iccl.2018.04.004
2211-7458/18/© 2018 Elsevier Inc. All rights reserved.

anatomic structures and their relationship to surrounding structures, or allow for virtual device testing. Application of 3D printing in structural heart interventions is not only filling a knowledge deficit of cardiac anatomy but also allowing more physicians to understand the anatomy as if they were working in a surgical field.

WHAT IS THREE-DIMENSIONAL PRINTING?

3D printing is a process of creation of a physical 3D model to be used for teaching, patient education, or device evaluation. The term 3D printing in medicine is a colloquial phrase for a process long-established in the architectural and manufacturing world as additive manufacturing or rapid prototyping.[3] 3D-printed models of patient specific anatomy can be generated from 3D transesophageal (TEE), cardiac MRI, or cardiac computed tomography (CT) datasets. CT datasets are most commonly used for accurate cardiac 3D printing given its thin-slice acquisition (0.625 mm) and ability to capture dynamic motion of the cardiac anatomy through both systole and diastole.

HOW TO PERFORM CARDIAC THREE-DIMENSIONAL PRINTING: FROM SCAN TO BENCHSIDE

After scan acquisition is completed, medical image datasets are stored in a format called Digital Imaging and Communications in Medicine (DICOM).[4,5] The DICOM format contains a large array of volumetric metadata that cannot be interpreted directly by 3D printers. 3D printers can interpret surface datasets, which consist of a meshwork made from triangles, not a volumetric dataset, which is the framework of medical imaging acquisition.[6]

For the 3D printer to be able to produce a final object, it must recognize which parts of the model are critical for the print and which parts are void (ie, space) that does not need to

be printed. With that, there is a certain degree of translation, interpretation, and proof that must occur to get from medical data to a final 3D model. This process is done via segmentation.[3,7] Segmentation of imaging generates multiple masks or objects for each part of the anatomy that can later be postprocessed to create a printable file (**Fig. 1**). These printable file formats are known as stereolithography (STL) or object files (OBJ). Both are surface files that contain information about positions of the individual triangles that make up the 3D model.

SELECTING THE IMAGING SOURCE DATA FOR THREE-DIMENSIONAL PRINTING

Although imaging can be acquired via multiple pathways (CT, MRI, or 3D TEE), not all imaging techniques are equivalent for the production of a 3D print. A dynamic dataset is typically optimal for cardiac 3D modeling because it has a temporal component that allows for the selection of the best phase (or cardiac cycle) to create an accurate model for a specific print.

Three-Dimensional Transesophageal Echocardiography Datasets

3D TEE datasets have a large quantity of information packed within a small timeframe. The high frequency of temporal acquisition allows for a large dataset (more than 100 volumes) between cardiac phases in systole and diastole.[8] This allows the clinician to narrow down the phase of the heartbeat of most interest for a 3D print evaluation. Compared with CT-derived datasets, 3D TEE datasets have poor temporal resolution because TEE has a narrower field of view and ultrasound waves have a limited ability to travel far distances.[8] Given these issues with the imaging display field of view, a 3D print generated by 3D TEE is limited to the structure of interest, which can create problems when multiple anatomies are needed for a model (**Fig. 2**). Examination of large surface anatomic interactions is not

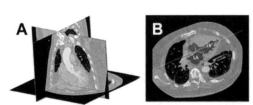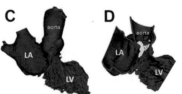

Fig. 1. The process of creating a model of the left heart/mitral annulus. (A) Images of the heart; (B) segmentation of the blood volume (*shown in red*); (C) 3D modeling of the chambers of the left heart; (D) Hollowed and sectioned model to view interior wall of left heart; (E) 3D printed model of the left heart (transapical view from the left ventricle looking into the mitral annulus). LA, left atrium; LV, left ventricle. (*Courtesy of* Janelle Schrot, Materialise NV, Leuven, Belgium.)

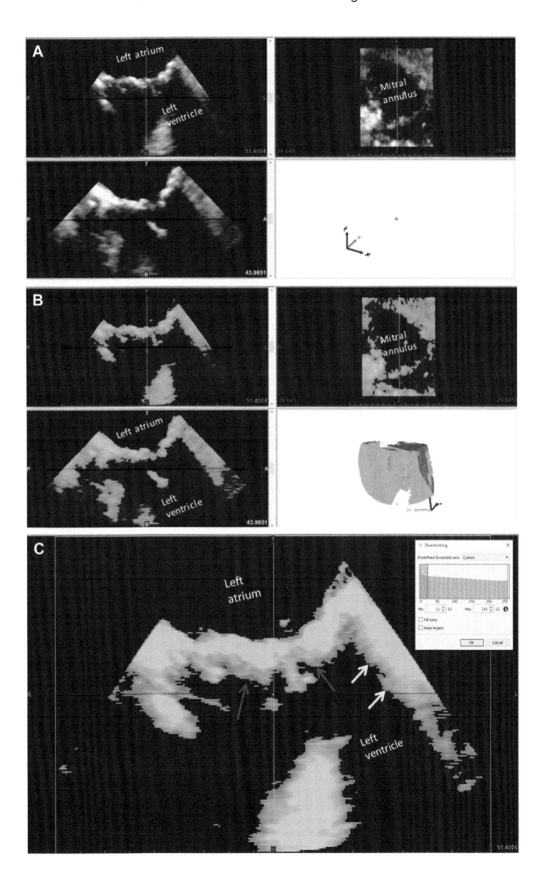

possible with current 3D TEE or surface echo technologies. Furthermore, most DICOM image datasets from 3D TEE are originally encoded in a proprietary format created by manufacturers (eg, Cartesian DICOM) that require an additional step to translate the data to standard DICOM format; adding to the difficulty of incorporating the application of 3D TEE for 3D printing into clinical workflow. Lastly, 3D TEE has a relatively narrow range of Hounsfield units that is presented during segmentation, which limits its application to 3D printing. Each anatomic part of the body, from bone to skin, tissue to blood, carries a different Hounsfield unit weight, that is applied in the segmentation process to distinguish fine anatomic structures. This limited window of Hounsfield unit differentiation in 3D TEE datasets decreases the accuracy of 3D TEE prints for sizing smaller structures. However, it remains reliable in gross localization of defects for transcatheter and surgical interventions. One of the most important advantages of 3D TEE is the availability of a nonradiation-dependent source of 3D imaging acquisition with little capital expenditure required for equipment (ie, it does not require CT scanner purchase or installation).

MRI Datasets

MRI for 3D printing has a different set of challenges. MRI scan acquisitions typically require patients to be able to lie flat and follow breath-holding commands intermittently for approximately 1 hour to allow a full cardiac MRI to be performed. Many structural heart patients, owing to their age, frailty, comorbidities, and existing internal mechanical devices, are not eligible for a cardiac MRI. If patients are able to tolerate a cardiac MRI, these datasets may be used for 3D printing. However, similar to 3D TEE, the MRI dataset has a small field of view and may not cover all of the anatomy of interest. Only very specific scans, such as the 3D full-phase navigated MRI, produce high-definition imaging that can be translated into a 3D print. Another limitation of MRI is slice thickness. MRI slices are quite thick ($\geq$3 mm), whereas traditional CT scans for the evaluation of transcatheter aortic valve replacement (TAVR) or transcatheter mitral

intervention are processed using slices equal to or less than 1.25 mm thick. This slice thickness could distort the final 3D print and potentially miss fine cardiac anatomic features.

Cardiac Computed Tomography Datasets

In the authors' experiences, cardiac CT datasets provide the best application for cardiac 3D printing. Multidetector CT allows for thin-slice (0.625 mm thickness) comprehensive noninvasive imaging of the cardiac anatomy and related structures. It provides reproducible quality and detailed anatomic information on size and function in an established DICOM format that can be efficiently converted to a printable file.[9–11]

However, cardiac CT has its own limitations. Given the use of radiation during scan image acquisition, this is unlikely to be the first noninvasive imaging modality of choice for the pediatric population. In patients with chronic renal insufficiency, a cardiac CT requiring at times equal to or greater than 80 cc of iodinated contrast may not be an option, and the use of a noncontrast CT for 3D cardiac modeling is limited. Hence, 3D TEE and cardiac MRI are being applied to 3D printing and planning for complex congenital heart cases in clinical practice.

Segmentation of 3D printing depends on accurately opacificying the anatomical structure of interest with contrast so softwares can assign a Hounsfield unit weight to that specific anatomy. The timing of the contrast bolus is critical for the adequacy of the 3D print and depends on the anatomic structure of interest. In TAVR CTs, the contrast bolus is timed to the descending aorta; in mitral and left atrial appendage (LAA) CTs, the contrast bolus is timed to the filling of the left atrium. In the adult population, care must be taken in segmentation to differentiate calcium deposits, heart myocardium, and valve leaflets. However, challenges may occur when CT scans do not have adequate contrast opacification due to contrast washout, or presence of artifacts from previous mechanical implants creating artificial artifacts and Hounsfield unit discrepancies (Fig. 3). These latter difficulties require manual override interpretation of automatic segmentation workflows to both

Fig. 2. Challenges in 3D printing from 3D transesophageal datasets. (A) 3D multi-planar dataset acquired from a 3D TEE DICOM file. (B) In green, thresholding of the myocardium and leaflets are attempted with a pre-defined Hounsfield Unit range. Thresholding of 3D TEE dataset (in green) demonstrating difficulty in delineating fine structures from coarse myocardium. (C) 3D TEE has a relatively narrow thresholding range for dataset segmentation which creates difficulty when trying to model different parts of the left ventricle (ie, leaflet in red arrow versus myocardium in yellow arrow). Note the narrow range of thresholding (box display) available for 3D TEE datasets, and bloomed over-amplification of anatomy secondary to narrow thresholding view.

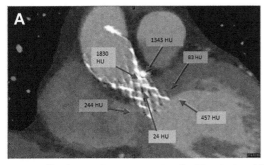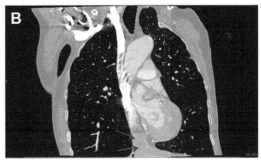

Fig. 3. Difficulties in CT segmentation for 3D printing. (A) Structures in close proximity in cardiac anatomy can have variable Housefield Unit uptake despite being adjacent to each other in a small confined 3D space. (B) Poor contrast filling (arrows) and washout in the lumen of the endovascular makes segmentation of CT difficult.

prevent the printing of incorrect structures and empty spaces when they clinically do not exist.

MEDICAL SOFTWARE

There are multiple free and commercial imaging segmentation software available for the creation of a 3D print. Selection of the software suite is critical to 3D laboratory efficiency and accuracy of the 3D print generated. Currently, the authors have found the Mimics Suite (Materialise, Leuven, Belgium) to be the most comprehensive medical computer-aided design (CAD) imaging segmentation software for 3D printing. Various free CAD toolkits are available; however, multiple softwares must be used to take a DICOM file from segmentation to STL file generation, to mesh model creation before final generation of a 3D print.[7] The latter level of complexity requires an industrial design background or engineering understanding of CAD and 3D printing software tools and capabilities.

THREE-DIMENSIONAL PRINTERS

There are many types of 3D printers. Selection of 3D printers primarily depends on the type of material the user wishes to print, the size of the print, and need for printing sterile implants. For small cardiac models, the Stratasys Objet 30pro (Stratasys, Eden Prairie, MN, USA) and the Formlabs Form1 printer (Formlabs, Somerville, MA, USA) are 2 entry-level 3D printers commonly found in hospitals with in-house 3D printing capabilities.

APPLICATIONS OF THREE-DIMENSIONAL PRINTING IN STRUCTURAL HEART INTERVENTIONS

The application of 3D printing technology offers several noteworthy advantages. First and foremost, it allows for personalized patient care with precise periprocedural planning. Second, 3D printing reduces intraprocedural guesswork regarding catheter and device selection, thus improving patient safety during structural heart interventions.[12] The graspable, 3D-generated model can be rotated and studied from all points of view to improve operator confidence in understanding the patient's pathologic condition and reduce the visual errors made from 2-dimensional (2D) images. By maneuvering the device and simulating implantation, new projections can be made that add to the information gathered from traditional imaging. The gained spatial resolution allows operators to foresee intraoperative complications and enables more precise planning.

Examples of common applications of 3D printing in structural heart interventions include the following.

Peri-valvular Leak Closure
3D printing plays an important role in helping localize the perivalvular defect requiring closure. 3D printing the anatomic location of interest also helps in selecting the appropriate angled or nonangled catheter to cross the perivalvular leak of interest (Fig. 4). This allows operators to minimize the amount of time spent in the catheterization laboratory searching for the defect, thereby minimizing extra contrast usage and radiation exposure to operators and patients during the case.

Left Atrial Appendage Closure
Application of 3D printing in LAA closure allows users to predefine the appropriate landing zone for different closure devices based on their shape and anticipated sealing of the LAA. The anatomy of the LAA has long been misunderstood as a very simple structure. A collage of 3D patient-specific LAAs demonstrates that the LAA is a unique anatomic structure in each person, akin to a fingerprint (Fig. 5). Predefining the angulations

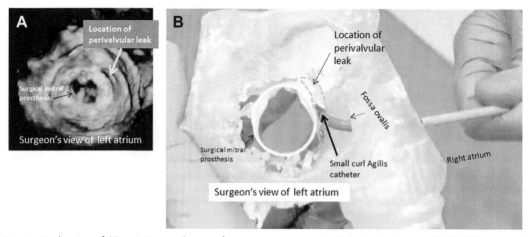

Fig. 4. Application of 3D printing in planning for percutaneous peri-valvular leak closure. (*A*) 3D TEE surgeon's view of antero-medial cresecent shaped peri-valvular defect (denoted by *yellow arrow*). (*B*) 3D print of the peri-valvular leak location to allow bench-testing for optimal catheter selection to cross the defect effectively.

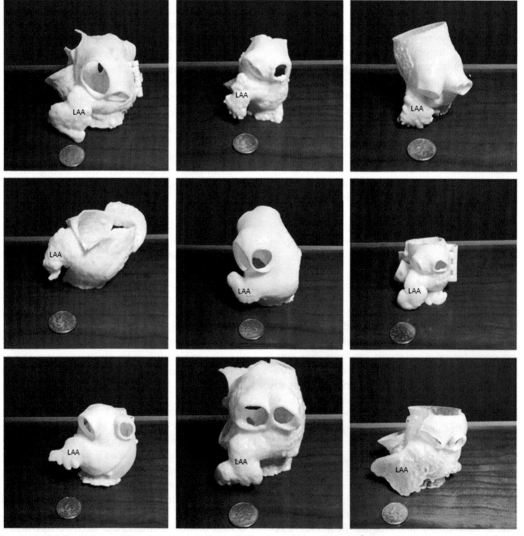

Fig. 5. Each left atrial appendage is unique. Collage of 3D printed left atrial appendages demonstrating each left atrial appendage is unique like a fingerprint, with different angulations and LAA ostium take-offs from the left atrium.

and size of patient-specific LAA closure by CT and 3D print has been shown in a prospective study to decrease the number of fluoroscopic angles, procedure times, and devices used for LAA closure with the WATCHMAN occluder (Boston Scientific, Marlborough, MA, USA).[13]

Transcatheter Mitral Valve Replacement

3D printing has changed the way physicians understand the mitral valve anatomy. With the increased awareness of risk of death with critical left ventricular outflow (LVOT) obstruction after transcatheter mitral valve replacement, 3D printing plays an integral role in teaching physicians to rethink the concept of the LVOT.[14,15] Implanting a virtual or physical valve in a virtual or physical 3D model allows physicians to optimize patient selection for candidacy for transcatheter

mitral interventions, and prevent inappropriate patient exclusions from clinical trials for patients due to inadequate 2D imaging technologies (**Fig. 6**).

COST OF THREE-DIMENSIONAL PRINTING

Cost is a major barrier to widespread adoption of 3D printing. Currently, Medicare does not have a reimbursement code for 3D printing, which further limits its use to academic investigators. Other barriers that exist also have to do with hospital cost centers. Often, CT and MRI are in the radiology cost center. However, structural heart interventions are becoming multidisciplinary, requiring the time of the radiologist, cardiologist, and 3D laboratory technologist. Thus, the professional and technical time

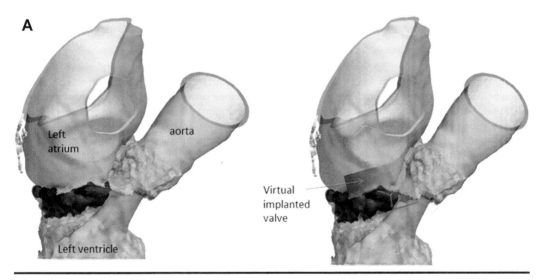

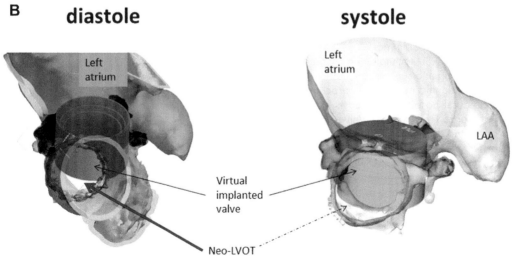

Fig. 6. (*A*) Traditional 2D TEE LVOT view of mitral annulus; (*B*) View from Aorta into left ventricle demonstrating LVOT obstruction occurring in mid to end-systole.

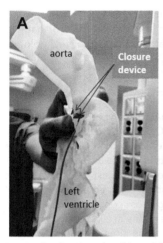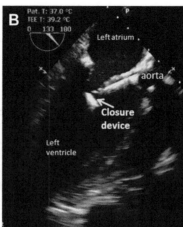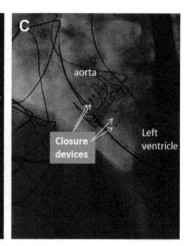

Fig. 7. Application of multi-modality imaging and 3D print in peri-valvular leak planning. (*A*) 3D printed model of the aorta and peri-valvular leak around the surgical aortic valve allows for bench test localization of the leak, and sizing of the leak with potential closure devices. (*B*) Intraprocedural 2D TEE demonstrating the closure device being exposed in the left ventricle prior to deployment across the peri-valvular leak. (*C*) Fluoroscopic overlay of the access obtained across the peri-valvular leak with multiple closure devices in place sealing the gap.

necessary to incorporate 3D printing into a structural heart program can lead to potential difficulties based on cost center and resource allocation. As modern medicine continues to become more integrative and interdisciplinary, this accounting issue will need to be addressed by health systems in an equitable manner.

SUMMARY

Solving a 3D problem using 2D tools has required the complementary use of multiple imaging modalities (**Fig. 7**). Understanding of the geometry, structure, and function of the heart is continuing to evolve. 3D prototyping has emerged as a promising periprocedural tool. 3D printing technology offers the promise of bridging the gap from 2D images on a screen to an accurate, graspable, and palpable model.[16]

By investing in 3D technology to optimize procedural planning and success, the authors predict there will be significant savings in procedural and postprocedural hospitalization costs. The Placement of Aortic Transcatheter Valves (PARTNER) trial offers the earliest insight into cost-effective analysis of structural heart procedures.[17] Much of the nonprocedural costs were dictated by length of stay and repeat hospitalizations. Improving the accuracy of a structural heart procedure will lead to more precise device sizing and safety of the procedure thereby impacting 2 drivers of the total cost of the procedure.

There are multiple advantages to 3D printing for patients, providers, and health systems. Patient education and disease awareness, especially in

those with repaired congenital heart disease, is an important tool in patient-centric engagement with their provider. Additionally, better procedural planning may lead to shorter procedural durations with lower radiation exposure. In turn, this can lead to more efficient utilization of procedural suites. This is an important consideration for health systems under pressure to generate profits with declining reimbursements.

At present, 3D printing does not solve all of the barriers in treating structural heart conditions. However, it will provide insights for investigators and clinicians into novel questions that have not been previously considered. Although 3D printing is currently in the innovation phase, it holds major promise for patients, clinicians, scientists, and hospital administrators to change the face of modern medicine. Clinical outcomes are related to a comprehensive understanding of a patient's anatomy.

ACKNOWLEDGMENTS

The authors wish to thank Tongwa Aka, Rewaa Yas, and Janelle Schrot for their help in the imaging preparation for this manuscript.

REFERENCES

1. Tack P, Victor J, Gemmel P, et al. 3D-printing techniques in a medical setting: a systematic literature review. Biomed Eng Online 2016;15(1):115.
2. Leon MB, Smith CR, Mack MJ, et al. Transcatheter or surgical aortic-valve replacement in intermediate-risk patients. N Engl J Med 2016;374(17):1609–20.

3. Mitsouras D, Liacouras P, Imanzadeh A, et al. Medical 3D printing for the radiologist. Radiographics 2015;35(7):1965–88.

4. Bidgood WD Jr, Horii SC, Prior FW, et al. Understanding and using DICOM, the data interchange standard for biomedical imaging. J Am Med Inform Assoc 1997;4(3):199–212.

5. Varma DR. Managing DICOM images: tips and tricks for the radiologist. Indian J Radiol Imaging 2012;22(1):4–13.

6. Ripley B, Levin D, Kelil T, et al. 3D printing from MRI Data: harnessing strengths and minimizing weaknesses. J Magn Reson Imaging 2017;45(3):635–45.

7. Bucking TM, Hill ER, Robertson JL, et al. From medical imaging data to 3D printed anatomical models. PLoS One 2017;12(5):e0178540.

8. Vegas A. Three-dimensional transesophageal echocardiography: principles and clinical applications. Ann Card Anaesth 2016;19(Supplement):S35–43.

9. Goldman LW. Principles of CT: multislice CT. J Nucl Med Technol 2008;36(2):57–68 [quiz: 75–6].

10. Nasis A, Mottram PM, Cameron JD, et al. Current and evolving clinical applications of multidetector cardiac CT in assessment of structural heart disease. Radiology 2013;267(1):11–25.

11. Ohnesorge B, Flohr T, Becker C, et al. Cardiac imaging by means of electrocardiographically gated multisection spiral CT: initial experience. Radiology 2000;217(2):564–71.

12. Wang DD, Eng M, Kupsky D, et al. Application of 3-dimensional computed tomographic image guidance to WATCHMAN implantation and impact on early operator learning curve: single-center experience. JACC Cardiovasc Interv 2016; 9(22):2329–40.

13. Eng MH, Wang DD, Greenbaum AB, et al. Prospective, randomized comparison of 3-dimensional computed tomography guidance versus TEE data for left atrial appendage occlusion (PRO3DLAAO). Catheter Cardiovasc Interv 2018. [Epub ahead of print].

14. Guerrero M, Wang DD, Himbert D, et al. Short-term results of alcohol septal ablation as a bail-out strategy to treat severe left ventricular outflow tract obstruction after transcatheter mitral valve replacement in patients with severe mitral annular calcification. Catheter Cardiovasc Interv 2017; 90(7):1220–6.

15. Wang DD, Eng MH, Greenbaum AB, et al. Validating a prediction modeling tool for left ventricular outflow tract (LVOT) obstruction after transcatheter mitral valve replacement (TMVR). Catheter Cardiovasc Interv 2017. [Epub ahead of print].

16. Michalski MH, Ross JS. The shape of things to come: 3D printing in medicine. JAMA 2014; 312(21):2213–4.

17. Reynolds MR, Magnuson EA, Lei Y, et al. Cost-effectiveness of transcatheter aortic valve replacement compared with surgical aortic valve replacement in high-risk patients with severe aortic stenosis: results of the PARTNER (Placement of Aortic Transcatheter Valves) trial (Cohort A). J Am Coll Cardiol 2012;60(25):2683–92.

Printed and bound by CPI Group (UK) Ltd, Croydon, CR0 4YY

03/10/2024

01040298-0017